SYSTEMIC LUPUS ERYTHEMATOSUS DIET COOKBOOK

Deliciously Simple SLE Recipes for Reducing Flare-Ups, Strengthening the Immune System, Maintaining Skin Health, and Preventing Autoimmune Disorders

Michael Slowick, RDN

COPYRIGHT PAGE

Copyright © 2024 Michael Slowick, RDN. All rights reserved.

No part of this publication or work may be copied, stored in a retrieval system, or transmitted in any form or by any means without prior written permission from the publisher or author, or through payment of the appropriate per-copy fee to the copyright holder, except as permitted under Sections 107 or 108 of the United States Copyright Act of 1976, or as expressly allowed by law, license, or terms agreed upon with the relevant reprographics rights organization.

The publisher and author expressly disclaim any implied guarantees of merchantability and fitness for a particular purpose. While every effort has been made to ensure the accuracy of the information provided herein, no promises are made regarding its completeness or accuracy. Any statements made by sales employees or representatives, whether verbal or written, do not constitute extended or implied guarantees.

Table of Contents

COPYRIGHT PAGE 2

Table of Contents 4

CHAPTER I: WHAT IS SYSTEMIC LUPUS ERYTHEMATOSUS (SLE)? 1

Types of SLE: Overview of different manifestations 9

Causes and triggers of SLE 11

Diagnosis and Treatment 14

Complications of Lupus 28

Impact of diet on SLE: How nutrition influences symptoms 30

CHAPTER II: NUTRITIONAL BASIS FOR MANAGING SLE 36

Anti-inflammatory diet principles 39

SLE diet Principles 43

Importance of hydration and its impact on SLE ... 50

CHAPTER III: DIETARY CONSIDERATIONS FOR SLE PATIENTS 58

Foods to avoid or limit: Triggers and exacerbating factors 62

Meal planning tips for SLE patients 66

CHAPTER 4: SAVORY RECIPES AND MEAL IDEAS FOR SYSTEMIC LUPUS ERYTHEMATOSUS (SLE) 71

SAVORY RECIPES AND MEAL IDEAS FOR BREAKFAST 71

Cinnamon porridge with baked bananas 71

Cinnamon twists 73

Banana & cinnamon pancakes with blueberry compote 77

Puff pastry cinnamon rolls 79

Salsa verde baked eggs 81

Sweetcorn fritters with eggs & black bean salsa ... 84

Nuts & seeds granola 87

Banana & cinnamon pancakes with blueberry compote 90

Almond crêpes with avocado & nectarines 92

Millet porridge with almond milk & berry compote 94

Berry omelette 96

Creamy smoked haddock & saffron kedgeree 98

Kale & salmon kedgeree 100

Cured salmon 102

SAVORY RECIPES AND MEAL IDEAS FOR LUNCH 107

Scandi trout with fennel potato salad 107

Tuna with peppery tomatoes & potatoes 109

Fresh salmon with Thai noodle salad 111

Spice-cured tuna tacos 114

Cheesy seafood bake 117

BBQ mackerel 120

Korean fishcakes with fried eggs & spicy salsa ... 122

Classic lasagne 125

Haddock in tomato basil sauce 129

Antipasti salmon 131

Sticky onion & cheddar quiche 134

Steamed bass with pak choi 137

Mackerel with orange & harissa glaze 139

Wild salmon with coconut chutney & green pilau 141

SAVORY RECIPES AND MEAL IDEAS FOR DINNER 145

Tomato & thyme cod 145

Creamy salmon, leek & potato traybake 147

Crushed new potato fish cakes with horseradish mayonnaise 149

Spicy Singaporean fish 152

Spiced fish & mussel pie 154

Spicy fish cakes with mango dipping sauce 157

One-pan Thai green salmon 161

Indian-spiced fish cakes 165

Tomato & mascarpone risotto 167

Mustard salmon & veg bake with horseradish sauce 169

Hake fish cakes with mustard middles 171

Baked sea bream with tomatoes & coriander 175

Herby fish fingers 177

Salmon & lemon mini fish cakes 179

SIDE DISH 182

Cheesy roasted courgettes 182

Baked feta with sesame & honey 183

Smoked haddock & cheddar fishcakes with watercress sauce 185

Lemon & coriander couscous 189

Perfect roast potatoes 190

Courgette & anchovy salad 192

Barbecued fennel with black olive dressing 194

Apricot pancakes with honey butter 196

Harissa cauliflower pilaf 198

Quinoa, pea & avocado salad 201

Spicy salmon tabbouleh 203

Warm mackerel & beetroot salad 206

Courgettes with mint & ricotta 208

Stir-fried greens with fish sauce 210

Fish o'leekie 211

Chapter 5: Lifestyle Strategies and Beyond For Managing SLE 214

Coping and support 214

Exercise and physical activity recommendations 216

Alternative therapies and their role in managing SLE 220

CHAPTER I: WHAT IS SYSTEMIC LUPUS ERYTHEMATOSUS (SLE)?

The immune system normally fights off dangerous infections and bacteria to keep the body healthy. An autoimmune disease occurs when the immune system attacks the body because it confuses it for something foreign. There are many autoimmune diseases, including systemic lupus erythematosus (SLE).

The term lupus has been used to identify a number of immune diseases that have similar clinical presentations and laboratory features, but SLE is the most common type of lupus. 70 % of people with lupus have it. It's what most people mean when they refer to "lupus".

SLE is a chronic disease that can have phases of worsening symptoms that alternate with periods of mild symptoms. SLE can cause inflammation of multiple organs or organ systems in the body, either acutely or chronically. In contrast, cutaneous lupus (CLE), is limited to the skin, although in some patients, it may eventually progress to SLE. Drug-induced lupus can be caused by certain prescription medications. It has many of the same symptoms as SLE but rarely affects major organs and disappears about six months after the medication is stopped. Neonatal lupus occurs only in newborns and is not true lupus. Most of the symptoms of neonatal lupus will disappear after six months.

Most people with SLE are able to live a normal life with treatment.

According to the Lupus Foundation of America, at least 1.5 million Americans are living with diagnosed lupus. The foundation believes that the number of people who actually have the condition is much higher and that many cases go undiagnosed.

What Causes Lupus?

The exact cause of lupus is unknown. However, studies have found that a combination of environmental, genetic, and hormonal factors play a role in its development. Lupus is not contagious.

A number of genes have been identified to be associated with lupus. People with these genes who are then exposed to certain environmental triggers may then develop lupus.

Environmental triggers such as ultraviolet B (UVB) radiation from the sun, certain infections like the Epstein-Barr virus, and toxins like cigarette smoke can alter the body's immune response when combined with genes associated with lupus.

Common environmental factors that are associated with the development of the disease and flares include:

- The sun

- Infections and other illnesses

- Exhaustion

- Emotional stress caused by events like illness, a death in the family, or divorce

- Physical stress caused by things like surgery, injury, pregnancy, or giving birth

- Sulfa drugs such as Bactrim and Septra (trimethoprim-sulfamethoxazole)

- Tetracycline drugs that make you more sun-sensitive, like Minocin (minocycline)

- Penicillin or other antibiotics

Women and Lupus

Women are more likely to develop lupus than men. Black women develop lupus more often than women of any other race.

Risk factors

Anyone can develop lupus, but some groups of people have a higher risk:

People assigned female at birth (AFAB), especially people AFAB between the ages of 15 and 44.

Black people.

Hispanic people.

Asian people.

Native Americans, Alaska Natives and First Nations people.

Pacific Islanders.

People with a biological parent who has lupus.

Symptoms

Lupus causes symptoms throughout your body, depending on which organs or systems it affects. Everyone experiences a different combination and severity of symptoms.

Lupus symptoms usually come and go in waves called flare-ups. During a flare-up, the symptoms can be severe enough to affect your daily routine. You might also have periods of remission when you have mild or no symptoms.

Symptoms of systemic lupus erythematosus (SLE) vary from person to person and they may come and go and change over time. Lupus shares symptoms with other diseases, which can make it difficult to diagnose. The most common symptoms include:

- Skin rashes

- Pain or swelling in the joints (arthritis)

- Swelling in the feet, and around the eyes (typically due to kidney involvement)

- Extreme fatigue

- Low fevers

Below is a brief description of some of the more serious complications of systemic lupus erythematosus involving major organ systems:

- Inflammation of the kidneys—called lupus nephritis—can affect the body's ability to filter waste from the blood. It can be so damaging that dialysis or a kidney transplant may be needed.

- Inflammation of the nervous system and brain can cause memory problems, confusion, headaches, and strokes.

- Inflammation in the brain's blood vessels can cause high fevers, seizures, and behavioral changes.

- Hardening of the arteries or coronary artery disease—the buildup of deposits on coronary artery walls—can lead to a heart attack.

- Inflammation of the skin can cause rashes, sores, and ulcers throughout the body. About half of all people with systemic lupus erythematosus will develop a malar rash — a butterfly-shaped rash mostly seen across the cheeks and nose that can get worse in the sunlight.

Types of SLE: Overview of different manifestations

There are four different types of lupus. Systemic lupus erythematosus (SLE) is the most common type of lupus. If SLE begins in childhood, it is known as childhood-onset SLE or cSLE. Approximately 10-20 percent of SLE cases begin in childhood. Most cases of SLE begin in adulthood, between the ages of 15-44. Lupus that only affects the skin is less common and is called cutaneous lupus erythematosus (CLE). There are three types of CLE – discoid lupus, subacute cutaneous lupus, and acute cutaneous lupus. Neonatal lupus and drug-induced lupus are the least common types of lupus.

- **Cutaneous lupus erythematous**: Lupus that only affects your skin.

- **Drug-induced lupus**: Some medications trigger lupus symptoms as a side effect. It's usually temporary and might go away after you stop taking the medication that caused it.

- **Neonatal lupus**: Babies are sometimes born with lupus. Babies born to biological parents with lupus aren't certain to have lupus, but they might have an increased risk.

How is SLE different from other forms of lupus?

SLE can cause inflammation of multiple organs or organ systems in the body, either acutely or chronically. In contrast, cutaneous lupus (CLE), is limited to the skin, although in some patients, it may eventually progress to SLE. Drug-induced lupus can be caused by certain prescription medications. It has many of the same symptoms as SLE but rarely affects major organs and disappears about six months after the medication is stopped. Neonatal lupus occurs only in newborns and is not true lupus. Most of the symptoms of neonatal lupus will disappear after six months.

Causes and triggers of SLE

Experts don't know what causes systemic lupus erythematosus, however, studies have found that a combination of environmental, genetic, and hormonal factors play a role in its development. Lupus is not contagious. A number of genes have been identified to be associated with lupus. People with these genes who are then exposed to certain environmental triggers may then develop lupus. The genetic mutations that researchers have associated with SLE often involve genes that regulate the body's immune function, which are called major histocompatibility complex (MHC) genes.

Not everyone with an SLE gene variation will develop the condition, however.

Environmental triggers such as ultraviolet B (UVB) radiation from the sun, certain infections like the Epstein-Barr virus, and toxins like cigarette smoke can alter the body's immune response when combined with genes associated with lupus.

Common environmental factors that are associated with the development of the disease and flares include:

- The sun

- Infections and other illnesses

- Exhaustion

- Emotional stress caused by events like illness, a death in the family, or divorce

- Physical stress caused by things like surgery, injury, pregnancy, or giving birth

- Sulfa drugs such as Bactrim and Septra (trimethoprim-sulfamethoxazole)

- Tetracycline drugs that make you more sun-sensitive, like Minocin (minocycline)

- Penicillin or other antibiotics

Women ages 15 to 44 and certain ethnic groups—including African American, Asian American, Hispanics/Latino, and Native American—are at higher risk for developing SLE than the rest of the population.

Diagnosis and Treatment

Diagnosis

Diagnosing lupus is difficult because signs and symptoms vary considerably from person to person. Signs and symptoms of lupus may change over time and overlap with those of many other disorders.

No one test can diagnose lupus. The combination of blood and urine tests, signs and symptoms, and physical examination findings leads to the diagnosis.

Laboratory tests

Blood and urine tests may include:

Complete blood count. This test measures the number of red blood cells, white blood cells and platelets as well as the amount of hemoglobin, a protein in red blood cells. Results may indicate you have anemia, which commonly occurs in lupus. A low white blood cell or platelet count may occur in lupus as well.

Erythrocyte sedimentation rate: This blood test determines the rate at which red blood cells settle to the bottom of a tube in an hour. A faster than normal rate may indicate a systemic disease, such as lupus. The sedimentation rate isn't specific for any one disease. It may be elevated if you have lupus, an infection, another inflammatory condition or cancer.

Kidney and liver assessment: Blood tests can assess how well your kidneys and liver are functioning. Lupus can affect these organs.

Urinalysis: An examination of a sample of your urine may show an increased protein level or red blood cells in the urine, which may occur if lupus has affected your kidneys.

Antinuclear antibody (ANA) test: A positive test for the presence of these antibodies — produced by your immune system — indicates a stimulated immune system. While most people with lupus have a positive antinuclear antibody (ANA) test, most people with a positive ANA do not have lupus. If you test positive for ANA , your doctor may advise more-specific antibody testing.

Imaging tests

If your doctor suspects that lupus is affecting your lungs or heart, he or she may suggest:

Chest X-ray: An image of your chest may reveal abnormal shadows that suggest fluid or inflammation in your lungs.

Echocardiogram: This test uses sound waves to produce real-time images of your beating heart. It can check for problems with your valves and other portions of your heart.

Biopsy

Lupus can harm your kidneys in many different ways, and treatments can vary, depending on the type of damage that occurs. In some cases, it's necessary to test a small sample of kidney tissue to determine what the best treatment might be. The sample can be obtained with a needle or through a small incision.

Skin biopsy is sometimes performed to confirm a diagnosis of lupus affecting the skin.

Lupus Treatment

Many treatment options are available to help you live well with lupus, although the condition is lifelong and has no cure. The goals are to reduce disease activity and minimize flares, prevent organ damage and further complications, and provide relief for pain and fatigue.

Nonsteroidal Anti-Inflammatory Drugs (NSAIDs)

Over-the-counter nonsteroidal anti-inflammatory drugs (NSAIDs), such as naproxen sodium (Aleve) and ibuprofen (Advil, Motrin IB, others), may be used to treat pain, swelling and fever associated with lupus. Stronger NSAIDs are available by prescription. Side effects of NSAIDs may include stomach bleeding, kidney problems and an increased risk of heart problems.

Antimalarial Drugs

Plaquenil (hydroxychloroquine, HCQ) and Aralen (chloroquine phosphate) are common antimalarial medications for treating lupus. HCQ has shown it can increase survival rates, reduce flares, and prevent organ damage. Although HCQ works by modulating the immune response, it does not make you immunocompromised and more susceptible to infection.

In rare cases, retinal toxicity or deposits on the retina (the light-sensing layer at the back of the eye) can occur. For this reason, people on HCQ will have their eye health monitored on a regular basis.

Corticosteroids

Prednisone and other types of corticosteroids can counter the inflammation of lupus. High doses of steroids such as methylprednisolone (Medrol) are often used to control serious disease that involves the kidneys and brain. Side effects include weight gain, easy bruising, thinning bones, high blood pressure, diabetes and increased risk of infection. The risk of side effects increases with higher doses and longer term therapy.

Immunosuppressants

Drugs that suppress the immune system may be helpful in serious cases of lupus. Examples include azathioprine (Imuran, Azasan), mycophenolate (Cellcept), methotrexate (Trexall, Xatmep, others), cyclosporine (Sandimmune, Neoral, Gengraf) and leflunomide (Arava). They can slow down or stop the immune response. They can treat lupus nephritis and complications with the central nervous system. They are usually for more severe cases of lupus. Potential side effects may include an increased risk of infection, liver damage, decreased fertility and an increased risk of cancer.

Biologics

Biologics such as Benlysta (belimumab) can target the body's immune system via injection or infusion. These medications can get expensive, but the drug companies that make them often have patient support programs to help you access them.

Side effects include nausea, diarrhea and infections. Rarely, worsening of depression can occur.

Rituximab (Rituxan, Truxima) may be beneficial for some people in whom other medications haven't helped. Side effects include allergic reaction to the intravenous infusion and infections.

In clinical trials, voclosporin has been shown to be effective in treating lupus.

Other potential drugs to treat lupus are currently being studied, including abatacept (Orencia), anifrolumab and others

Other Medications

Medications for treating other diseases that are linked to lupus may also help with symptoms. These medications can include things like drugs to treat high blood pressure or osteoporosis (progressive bone thinning).

Lupus Self-Care

Though treatments work to control disease activity and reduce the amount and severity of flares, living well with lupus also requires a certain amount of personal responsibility for your own health.

Self-care for lupus is about learning to live in your new normal in a way that makes sense to you. Although self-care will look different for everyone, here are some things to think about as you discover what you need to do to take care of yourself.

Give Yourself Permission to Grieve

Adjusting to life with a chronic illness is hard. You may find yourself mourning the life you used to have, and that's OK. Allow yourself to grieve.

Give yourself permission to be angry or sad. Just because you get an official diagnosis doesn't mean you have to accept it right away. It will take time to adjust to your new normal.

Find Ways to Conserve Energy

Fatigue affects most people with lupus and can have a significant effect on their quality of life. You may find that you only have a certain amount of energy every day. When that energy is gone, you may have nothing left to give.

In this case, self-care may look like altering simple tasks. For example, put a chair in the shower if washing your hair worsens your fatigue. Sit down to get dressed or put on makeup. Buy cut vegetables or ask a friend to help prepare meals.

Learn to Say No

Not everyone will understand what you're going through or how lupus affects you. Lupus is often an invisible disease.

No one can tell how fatigued you are or how much pain you are feeling. It's OK to say no to happy hour with friends or taking on an extra task at work if you know it will worsen your symptoms. The more you tell people what you are going through, the more easily they will understand your challenges.

Find a Support Group

You don't have to face lupus alone. There are many online and in-person support groups in which you can talk to other people who are going through the same things you are.

How to Reduce Lupus Flare-Ups

Lupus flares, or periods when symptoms worsen or reappear, can be overwhelming, especially if you've been in a period of remission.

A flare often feels like you're getting sick again. You may experience similar symptoms that you experienced when you were first diagnosed, or you may experience new symptoms. Taking steps to reduce flares can help you manage the disease.

Avoid the Sun

The sun is a major trigger for lupus flares. Avoid being outdoors during peak sun hours—10 a.m. to 3 p.m. If you must be in the sun, seek shade and wear sunscreen and sun-protective clothing.

Maintain Good Health

People with lupus are more susceptible to infections and illnesses, which can trigger flares. Try to avoid others who are sick and wash your hands often.

Get regular exercise that is appropriate for you and your symptoms, practice good sleep hygiene, and find ways to reduce stress. If you smoke, stop.

Stay Compliant With Treatments

A healthcare provider creates a treatment plan with the goals of reducing flares and preventing further complications and organ damage. Even if you are feeling better, stick to your treatment plan.

People who stop taking hydroxychloroquine are at a higher risk of flares.

Get regular exercise

Exercise can help keep your bones strong, reduce your risk of heart attack and promote general well-being.

Don't smoke

Smoking increases your risk of cardiovascular disease and can worsen the effects of lupus on your heart and blood vessels.

Eat a healthy diet

A healthy diet emphasizes fruits, vegetables and whole grains. Sometimes you may have dietary restrictions, especially if you have high blood pressure, kidney damage or gastrointestinal problems.

Ask your doctor if you need vitamin D and calcium supplements

There is some evidence to suggest that people with lupus may benefit from supplemental vitamin D. A calcium supplement can help you meet the daily recommended dietary allowance of 1,000 milligrams to 1,200 milligrams — depending on your age — to help keep your bones healthy.

Complications of Lupus

Between one-third and one-half of people living with lupus experience inflammation that affects their kidneys, resulting in a condition called lupus nephritis. Without treatment, lupus nephritis can progress to end-stage renal disease, which is a life-threatening condition.

Lupus nephritis causes the following symptoms:

- painful or swollen joints

- muscle pain

- fever

- a butterfly-shaped rash on the face

SLE can affect the heart, leading to inflamed tissue around this organ and abnormal heart valves, among other issues. Atherosclerosis, a form of heart disease, is more common among people with SLE than among those who do not have this condition. Pericarditis is a swelling of the membrane around the heart that can cause pain in the chest and shortness of breath

SLE can damage the nervous system and contribute to the following conditions:

- weakness in the limbs

- changes in sensations

- difficulty processing thoughts

- seizures

- stroke

Pleuritis (pleurisy) is inflammation of the lining of the lungs. It can cause shortness of breath and difficulty exercising.

These complications do not happen to everyone with lupus but can occur.

Impact of diet on SLE: How nutrition influences symptoms

Carbohydrates

Carbohydrates are among the macronutrients that provide energy and, when consumed in excess, contribute to increased energy storage and subsequent weight gain. Although there is no clear evidence that altering the proportion of total carbohydrate in the diet is an important determinant of energy intake, nutritional imbalance, and excess carbohydrate dietary intake have been suggested as risk factors that exacerbate clinical manifestations of several autoimmune diseases such as rheumatoid arthritis and SLE.

Obesity is a well-known risk factor for low-grade inflammation characterized by activation of several pathways involved in the expression of inflammatory cytokines such as tumor necrosis factor-alpha (TNF-α) and interleukin (IL)-6. Activation of these proinflammatory pathways significantly contributes to the perpetuation of the inflammatory response, which are at least partly responsible for the severe co-morbidities seen in SLE patients.

Obesity has a strong impact on organism functioning and is linked to the development of all diseases of civilization. Strong evidence also links obesity to many autoimmune disorders including SLE. Obesity in SLE patients is associated with a poorer outcome, higher disease activity and higher cumulative organ damage.

Proteins

The restriction of dietary protein has been addressed in several studies in patients with SLE and animal models. These data should be interpreted in a wider context as diet composition rather than protein restriction alone may show beneficial effects on SLE course. As an example, a traditional Mediterranean diet provides protection from certain chronic diseases including autoimmune disorders. This diet consists of vegetables, fruits, nuts, grains, olive oils and fish with limited meat consumption. Reduction of protein intake may be a reasonable approach in cases of lupus nephropathy as high protein intake contributes to reduced renal filtration, directly leading to the progression of kidney damage.

It has also been postulated that not only proteins but also selected amino acids may influence the course of SLE.

Essential Fatty Acids

Fatty acids (FAs), especially polyunsaturated FAs (PUFAs), are an effective and essential dietary factor for patients with SLE. Among PUFAs, omega-3 (ω-3) fatty acids [i.e., docosahexaenoic acid (DHA) and eicosapentaenoic acid (EPA)] can reduce the level of inflammatory mediators as well as CRP.

Despite certain fatty acids significantly improving SLE conditions, some research has indicated ambiguity concerning their effectiveness in SLE (especially of ω-3 and ω-6 PUFAs), which are related to overconsumption, dose-dependent complexity, adverse immune responses and accelerated autoimmune symptoms; these should be carefully considered.

Fiber

Dietary fiber consists of edible carbohydrate polymers with three or more monomeric units that are resistant to endogenous digestive enzymes and are thus neither hydrolysed nor absorbed in the small intestine. Although fiber is present in a wide range of plant-based food sources, consumption is low in Western countries, contributing to changes in gut microbiota that may influence the development of serious gastrointestinal, cardiovascular and autoimmune disorders.

Therefore, an adequate intake of dietary fiber is recommended in patients with SLE because of the beneficial effects of fiber in reducing the disease activity by decreasing serum levels of autoantibodies and inflammatory cytokines.

CHAPTER II: NUTRITIONAL BASIS FOR MANAGING SLE

Autoimmune diseases are characterized by chronic inflammation, where the immune system remains perpetually active, leading to tissue damage. The underlying causes of autoimmune diseases are complex, involving genetic, environmental, and hormonal factors. Diet, an environmental factor, is important as it can either exacerbate or alleviate inflammation. Inflammation is the body's natural response to injury or infection, but in autoimmune diseases, this response becomes chronic. Certain foods can influence inflammatory pathways. For instance, omega-3 fatty acids found in fish oil have anti-inflammatory properties, whereas trans fats and high sugar intake can promote inflammation.

The Role of diet in autoimmune disease management

Anti-inflammatory diets: These diets focus on reducing foods that trigger inflammation and incorporating those with anti-inflammatory properties. A prominent example is the Mediterranean diet, rich in fruits, vegetables, whole grains, lean protein, and healthy fats like olive oil. Studies have shown that this diet can reduce markers of inflammation and improve symptoms in conditions like rheumatoid arthritis and IBD.

Gluten-free diet: Gluten, a protein found in wheat, barley, and rye, can exacerbate symptoms in certain autoimmune conditions, particularly celiac disease and some cases of Hashimoto's thyroiditis. For these patients, a strict gluten-free diet can lead to significant symptom improvement and even remission.

Paleo diet: This diet emphasizes eating whole, unprocessed foods similar to what our ancestors might have eaten, including meat, fish, vegetables, fruits, nuts, and seeds. The elimination of processed foods, dairy, and grains aims to reduce inflammation and support a healthier immune system. Some individuals with autoimmune diseases report reduced symptoms and better overall health on a Paleo diet.

Specific Carbohydrate Diet (SCD): Particularly used for managing IBD, SCD eliminates complex carbohydrates that are believed to feed harmful bacteria in the gut. By reducing these bacteria, the diet aims to reduce gut inflammation and improve digestion.

Nutrient-rich foods: Certain nutrients play a pivotal role in immune function. Vitamin D, for instance, modulates the immune response and has been linked to reduced risk and severity of autoimmune diseases. Omega-3 fatty acids from fish, flaxseeds, and walnuts can also help lower inflammation. Antioxidant-rich foods like berries, dark leafy greens, and nuts combat oxidative stress, which can exacerbate autoimmune conditions.

Anti-inflammatory diet principles

The idea behind an anti-inflammatory diet is that the foods you eat may help with inflammation in the body and help lower the risks of diseases associated with chronic inflammation.

There's no one way to follow an anti-inflammatory diet. You can mix it up and tailor the eating plan to your family's tastes and needs. That said, there are some guidelines that you can follow on an anti-inflammatory diet:

• Eat five to nine servings of antioxidant-rich fruits and vegetables each day.

• Replace red meat with lean poultry, fish, beans, and lentils.

• Swap margarine and butter for health-promoting fats like olive oil.

• Reduce your intake of refined grains like white bread, saltines, and pastries, and choose more fiber-rich whole grains like oats, quinoa, brown rice, and pasta.

- Use anti-inflammatory herbs like garlic, ginger, and turmeric instead of seasoning your meals with salt.

- Do not deep fry your food—opt for baked, boiled, or braised cooking instead.

Benefits of an Anti-Inflammatory Diet

Certain foods are known to contribute to inflammation in the body. One example is red meat, which contains a lot of saturated fat—one of the substances (along with trans fat and refined sugar) that cause immune cells to release inflammatory proteins into the bloodstream.

On the other hand, while more research is needed, it's believed that eating an anti-inflammatory diet lowers the risk for these and other health conditions linked to inflammation.

- Obesity and metabolic disorder

- Heart disease

- Diabetes

- Cancer

- Arthritis

- Chronic obstructive pulmonary disease (COPD)

- Inflammatory bowel disease

- Alzheimer's and dementia

In one study, following an anti-inflammatory diet for one year led to a 37% decrease in inflammatory substances in the blood (such as C-reactive protein) in people with type 2 diabetes. Other studies looking at different variations of the anti-inflammatory diet, such as vegetable-rich diets or seafood-rich diets, have shown similar benefits, especially in people with heart disease.

In general, anti-inflammatory foods are rich in substances called antioxidants that fight chemicals (free radicals) that cause long-term damage to cells and can increase inflammation in the body.

SLE diet Principles

Healthy eating can make a big difference in your lupus symptoms and your overall health. It can also help prevent or manage other health conditions you may have, like high blood pressure or diabetes. There's no special "lupus diet" you need to follow — just work on building a balanced diet with healthy foods you enjoy.

Eat a variety of healthy foods

Eating a variety of healthy foods can give your body the nutrition it needs to manage your symptoms. Follow these tips:

- Eat lots of fruits and vegetables — try to make half your plate fruits and veggies

- Choose whole grains — like whole-wheat bread and pasta, oatmeal, and brown rice

- Get a mix of healthy proteins — like lean meats, poultry, seafood, beans, nuts, and eggs

- Go for foods with healthy fats — like olive oil, avocados, nuts, and fish

If you have lupus nephritis (a kidney disease caused by lupus), you may need to limit certain foods.

If you need help making healthy food choices, talk with your doctor — they can refer you to a registered dietician (a doctor who specializes in nutrition).

Can I be vegetarian or vegan if I have lupus?

Yes — it's fine for people with lupus to eat a vegetarian or vegan diet. Just make sure to eat a variety of healthy plant-based foods. If you don't eat any animal foods, you'll need to take a vitamin B12 supplement — vitamin B12 is only found in animal foods.

Are there any specific foods I need to avoid?

According to Johns Hopkins Lupus Center experts, they believe that a chemical found in alfalfa may trigger lupus symptoms. So you may want to avoid eating alfalfa sprouts or taking supplements with alfalfa.

You may also see claims that certain foods like garlic cause inflammation, but there is no scientific evidence to support this. If you have lupus and notice an increase in your lupus symptoms after consuming garlic or any other food, you should discuss this with your doctor.

Get key nutrients for bone and heart health

Lupus raises your risk for heart disease and osteoporosis (a bone disease that makes bones more likely to break). The good news is that eating healthy can help lower your risk.

For bone health, eat foods with lots of calcium, including:

- Leafy greens — like spinach and kale

- Dairy foods — like milk, yogurt, and soy milk

- Whole-grain cereals fortified with calcium

For heart health, eat foods with Omega-3 fatty acids, including:

- Fatty fish — like salmon, mackerel, and sardines

- Nuts and seeds — like walnuts and flax seeds

Do I need to take supplements?

Some people with lupus need supplements to get enough of certain nutrients, like vitamin D. But supplements can interact with your lupus medicines, so it's important to always talk with your doctor before you start taking any supplements.

Limit sodium, saturated fat, and added sugars

Cutting down on these 3 things can lower your risk for serious health problems like high blood pressure and diabetes — or help you manage these conditions. And small changes in your eating habits can make a big difference!

Cut down on sodium

Eating too much sodium (salt) can raise your risk for high blood pressure, which can cause heart attack and stroke. You could have high blood pressure and not know it — so it's important to limit sodium to keep your blood pressure in a healthy range. Try these tips:

• Cook more meals at home — packaged foods and restaurant meals are often high in sodium

• Check the Nutrition Facts label on packaged foods, and choose options with less sodium

• Flavor your food with herbs and spices instead of salt

Switch to healthier fats

Eating too much saturated fat (the kind of fat in animal foods like fatty meats and dairy) can raise your risk for heart disease and diabetes. And replacing saturated fat with healthier unsaturated fats can lower your risk. Try these tips:

- Cook with olive oil instead of butter

- Have fish or chicken as a protein instead of fatty meats like ribs or sausage

- Choose lower-fat dairy, like skim or nonfat milk and yogurt

Skip added sugars

Avoiding added sugars can also help prevent or manage conditions like heart disease and diabetes. There's a lot of added sugars in packaged foods and drinks like cookies and soda — but honey, sugar, and syrups that you add to foods and drinks at home count, too. Try these tips:

- Drink water instead of sugary soda — try adding herbs or fresh fruit to sparkling water for extra flavor

- Eat fruit for dessert instead of sugary treats like cake or ice cream

- Try drinking your coffee and tea without sugar — or add just 1 teaspoon

Do I need to limit alcohol?

If you drink alcohol, it's important to drink only in moderation — that means one drink or less in a day. Alcohol can also interact with some lupus medicines, including blood thinners. Ask your doctor if you need to avoid alcohol with your medicines.

Importance of hydration and its impact on SLE

Dehydration is bad for everyone, but people with lupus are especially vulnerable to the symptoms. Aside from feeling thirsty, there are other signs of dehydration, including:

- Dark colored urine

- Dry mouth

- Dry eyes

- Fatigue or sleepiness

- Headaches

- Confusion

- Dizziness or lightheadedness

At serious levels of dehydration, people will produce little to no urine, sweat, or tears. This is very severe and requires extreme treatment. Don't get to this point.

People with lupus have to keep an eye on their hydration more than most, especially if they have kidney trouble, as in lupus nephritis. And even more so if they also have Sjogren's syndrome, an autoimmune disease that affects the glands that produce saliva, mucous, and tears. People with

Sjogrens syndrome need to drink more water to make up for their decreased production, reduce their symptoms, and avoid dehydration.

Temperature and air quality can also contribute to dehydration. People with lupus are particularly sensitive to cold weather, hot weather, and humidity, which all effect how the body loses or holds water. Heat causes more water to be lost through sweat and breathing as the body tries to cool itself. Humid weather such as hot and muggy summer days can lead to overheating, which can trigger flares.

For people with lupus specifically, however, proper hydration can reduce inflammation by encouraging a healthier immune system. Hydration also keeps the kidneys healthy, reducing symptoms and the risk of kidney damage. It also improves mouth and tooth health, which are common issues for people with lupus.

Tips and Tricks to Staying Hydrated

Drinking plain water, is generally considered to be the best. If there is safe tap water, then that water is just as good as bottled water. Juices, milk, and herbal teas are second best, though you should watch out for sugar intake. Sugar can exacerbate inflammation and is just something to be careful about in general. Keep a water bottle with you and keep refilling it when it gets low. Because the body takes a while to register that it needs water, you should drink from it regularly, even when not thirsty. A common adage is "drink 8 cups of water per day," and if that helps you stay hydrated, then go for it. Drink on a schedule if that helps.

If plain or cold water is not working for you, warm water or tea might be what you need. You can also get a lot of water from your food, especially fruits and vegetables. These are mostly water and will also provide electrolytes and other nutrients. Including these in your diet will help with hydration and overall health. Read more about diets and lupus here. Caffeinated beverages, including green tea, do provide some water, though they can cause jitteriness and encourage urination.

If you have been exercising and sweating a lot, or are having trouble quenching your thirst, then electrolyte-containing beverages such as sports drinks can help. Electrolytes are minerals that are dissolved in the fluids of your body. They are important for many life functions and include sodium, calcium, potassium, chlorine, phosphate, and magnesium. When kept in balance with each other in the body, alongside water, electrolytes keep the organs and bloodstream healthy. The levels in the body are managed by the kidneys and skin, as well as by one's diet.

Because they help the body hold onto and better use water, electrolytes help quench the sensation of thirst and maintain a healthy level of hydration. However, sports drinks also often contain sugars, salts, and caffeine that you can't control. These can have negative effects on one's health, especially for people with lupus.

However, there are easier, healthier, (and cheaper) ways to make an electrolyte-rich beverage. Vinegar diluted in water with a small amount of sugar is a simple recipe that is easily controlled and effective. Other acidic fruits, such as lemons or limes, also provide electrolytes and add flavor to water. These fruit-based options are acidic, however, so lupuswarriors with tooth or GI problems should be careful. However, they also contain vitamin C, which is an antioxidant that plays a large role in how the body heals itself.

Alcohol is very bad at hydrating. In fact, part of the cause of hangovers is from dehydration! What water it provides is mostly urinated out as the body tries to flush the alcohol from the system. This is why many hangover remedies involve electrolytes – you are quickly rehydrating the body!

Changing one's environment can help, too: stay cool on hot days and use humidifiers on cool days. Humidifiers can help prevent drying out, which can help avoid dehydration.

Fluid Retention and Lupus

Many people with lupus have issues with water retention and swelling, particularly in their abdomens, legs, and ankles. When electrolytes are out of balance due to inflammation or kidney damage, then the body starts to retain water to try to maintain a balance. This causes swelling and can be embarrassing and uncomfortable. Water retention can also be caused by antimalarial medications such as Plaquenil, which are often used in lupus. Steroidal medications such as prednisone also cause fluid retention in the body.

The answer is to drink more water and adjust the diet – in particular focusing on reducing salt and increasing Vitamin B6, magnesium, and potassium intake. The medications may make it difficult for the body to manage its water balance, but remaining hydrated and reducing the electrolytes in the bloodstream makes it less likely to hold onto its water. Non-steroidal anti-inflammatory medications (NSAIDs) can also help with swelling caused by water retention.

CHAPTER III: DIETARY CONSIDERATIONS FOR SLE PATIENTS

What to Eat

It is a good idea to include a variety of fruits and vegetables, low calorie and low-fat foods, and foods high in antioxidants, fiber, calcium, vitamin D, and omega-3 fatty acids to your lupus diet. Having a healthy balance is important—that is, not eating too much of one thing or too little of another.

Compliant Foods

- Fish

- Fruits and vegetables

- Plant sources of omega-3 fatty acids (walnuts, flaxseeds, legumes)

- Whole grains

- Yogurt and dairy

Non-Compliant Foods

- Alfalfa sprouts

- Garlic

- Nightshade vegetables

- Processed or refined foods

- Alcohol

- Salt

Because lupus is an inflammatory condition, it is possible foods that fight off inflammation can reduce lupus symptoms. Some top anti-inflammatory foods to add to your diet include:

Fish: Omega-3 fatty acids—eicosapentaenoic acid (EPA) and docosahexaenoic acid (DHA)—are found in fatty fish, including salmon, sardines, and tuna. EPA and DHA can reduce inflammation that leads to numerous medical conditions, including heart disease and inflammatory arthritis. Studies have shown people who consume salmon or EPA and DHA supplements experience reductions in C-reactive markers—proteins responsible for inciting inflammation in the body. Aim to eat fatty fish at least twice a week to enjoy its anti-inflammatory effects.

Fruits and vegetables: Colorful produce—spinach, lettuce, carrots, blueberries, oranges, and more—are loaded with contain antioxidants and polyphenols—natural plant compounds to fight inflammation. Aim for at least five servings a day from a range of colors.

Vegetarian omega-fatty acids. Plant sources of omega-3 fatty acids—walnuts, flaxseeds, kidney beans, soybean oil, edamame, and more—contain alpha-linolenic acid (ALA). The body converts ALA to EPA and DHA. While the process is slow, you can still get some anti-inflammatory benefits from eating foods containing ALA.

Whole grains: People with lupus should aim to eat whole grains instead of refined ones. Whole-grain options to include in a lupus-friendly diet include rice, barley, bulgur (cracked wheat), oatmeal, quinoa, and whole-grain breads, pasta, and/or cereals.

Yogurt and dairy: Research shows a type of healthy bacteria found in yogurt and other dairy products might reduce disease symptoms in some people with lupus. In addition, eating foods high in calcium and vitamin D is important for people with lupus because they have an increased risk for osteoporosis. When buying dairy products, pick ones that are low-fat or fat-free. If you cannot drink milk, good alternatives are lactose-free, soy, and almond milk, and juice fortified with calcium and vitamin D.

Foods to avoid or limit: Triggers and exacerbating factors

Foods to Avoid

There are some foods that may trigger flare-ups of lupus symptoms. It should be noted, however, that the research on any specific connection between these foods and lupus is limited.

Some foods that may increase lupus symptoms are:

Alfalfa: Some research has linked alfalfa sprouts to lupus flares. This is because of a compound called L-canavanine that accelerates the immune system. Some studies have revealed eating alfalfa sprouts can induce a lupus-like syndrome in people who don't have lupus or reactivate lupus in people with inactive disease. If eating alfalfa sprouts induces a lupus flare for you, it may be a good idea to avoiding eating them.

Garlic: There has been evidence suggesting people with lupus should avoid garlic. Garlic contains three ingredients—allicin, ajoene, and thiosulfinate—that can amp up the immune system and cause an overactive response in people with lupus. Of course, eating small amounts of garlic will not hurt you, but it may help to limit the amount in your diet.

Processed and refined foods: Examples of processed foods are ones that come in a box or a can. These foods are often higher in fat, sugar, and salt. Refined foods, including white bread, pastas, and rice, also contain high amounts of fat, sugar, and salt. Studies show diets high in processed and refined foods can increase inflammation throughout the body. You should replace these types of foods with ones containing fresher and healthier ingredients, especially if you notice any increase in lupus symptoms after consuming them.

Nightshade vegetables: For some people with inflammatory conditions, including lupus, when eating nightshade vegetables—tomatoes, eggplant, peppers, etc.—they see an increase in inflammation. However, the Lupus Foundation of American notes there is no solid evidence to support this claim. Nonetheless, if nightshade vegetables increase your symptoms, you may want to remove them from your diet.

Alcohol: You do not have to give up drinking altogether. It is OK to have a glass of wine or beer every once in a while. But you should not drink too much alcohol because it may interfere with the medications you are taking to treat lupus. According to the Lupus Foundation of America, people with lupus who take certain drugs should avoid alcohol because of the risk for specific alcohol-medication interactions. For example, medications like methotrexate, a commonly prescribed medication for lupus, are metabolized in the liver and mixing them with alcohol could increase your risk for irreversible liver problems. Other drugs, such as prednisone and non-steroidal anti-inflammatory drugs (NSAIDs), when mixed with alcohol further increase the risk for gastrointestinal bleeding.

Salt: Eating too much salt isn't good for anyone and especially people with chronic health conditions like lupus. Excessive salt consumption can also increase the risk of high blood pressure and heart disease. But reducing salt intake doesn't have to be tasteless. You can substitute salt with herbs, such as mint and basil, spices, including cinnamon or pepper, or other foods, such as lemon to add great taste to food.

Meal planning tips for SLE patients

Cooking Tips

Cooking and eating at home can help you to avoid fast foods and meals that are loaded with saturated fats. While cooking at home, here are some things to keep in mind while you plan and prepare meals:

Use healthy fats: Fat is not always bad for you and it helps add taste to your foods. Just make sure you are picking unsaturated fats—such as olive oil, avocados, or nuts—over saturated fats like butter and margarine.

Limit sugar and salt: Eating too much sugar or salt can over time put you at additional risk for lupus co-morbidities, such as heart disease and high blood pressure. Make sure you are checking labels and using salt or sugar sparingly as you prepare meals. Use herbs, spices, vinegar, or lemon over salt.

Try global flavors: Some of the healthiest dishes come from the Mediterranean and countries like Japan, Thailand, and China and are rich in vegetables and whole grains. They also use spices like curry powder and herbs like ginger that not only add great flavor but are also known for their anti-inflammatory properties. You will want to use herbs and spices sparingly, as overconsumption of some of these may cause gastrointestinal symptoms.

Plan meals: Meal planning can make it easier for you to make healthy choices and set you up for success as you work towards managing lupus symptoms. It does not matter what your meal planning looks like as long as you make a plan and stick to it. And as you prepare meals, choose whole grains over refined grains, and smaller portions of leaner meats or vegetable proteins. You will also want to fill your plate with healthy vegetables.

Be mindful: Choose vegetables and fresh fruits whenever possible. Or sauté foods with healthy oils instead of deep-frying. You should also have some idea of what healthy portion sizes look like, so you don't end up eating more than you had planned.

Modifications

The diet choices you make with lupus cannot be successful if you are not managing other aspects of your life with lupus. This can include things like spacing out meals, not smoking, supplementing vitamin D if needed, staying active, getting enough rest, and keeping your stress levels low.

Space out meals: If you find you are having gastrointestinal symptoms, such as indigestion, you may want to try eating four or five smaller meals, instead of three large ones. Additionally, because fat is difficult to digest for people with lupus, you may want to avoid high-fat meals.

Avoid smoking: Smoking is known for complicating and accelerating the effects of lupus. It can also lower the effectiveness of the medications you take to treat lupus. If you need help quitting, talk to our healthcare provider about the best ways to accomplish this.

Supplement with vitamin D: Lupus, much like other autoimmune diseases, is associated with low levels of vitamin D. If you aren't spending enough time outdoors, you may want to talk to your healthcare provider about getting your levels tested and whether you need a vitamin D supplement.

Stay active: In addition to diet, gentle forms of physical activity can help you to manage lupus symptoms. Try brisk walking, swimming, water aerobics, biking, or using an elliptical machine or treadmill. Commit to at least one activity every day.

Get enough rest: Make sure you are making sleep a priority and trying to get seven to nine hours of sleep every night. You should also take breaks throughout your day to unwind and rest.

Manage stress: Emotional stress and other daily challenges can trigger lupus flares. By finding ways to relax, you can keep your stress levels in check.

CHAPTER 4: SAVORY RECIPES AND MEAL IDEAS FOR SYSTEMIC LUPUS ERYTHEMATOSUS (SLE)

SAVORY RECIPES AND MEAL IDEAS FOR BREAKFAST

Cinnamon porridge with baked bananas

Ingredients

- 80g porridge oats

- 150ml semi-skimmed milk

- ½ tsp ground cinnamon

- 1 large ripe banana (120g), halved lengthways and cut in half

- ½ orange, zested and juiced

- 200g plain bio yogurt

- 2 tsp toasted three-seed mix

Instructions

- STEP 1

Put the oats, milk, 450ml water and cinnamon in a pan. Bring to the boil, then turn the heat to low, stirring often, for 5 mins until thickened.

- STEP 2

Meanwhile, put the bananas in a dish with the orange zest and juice. Cover and microwave on high for 1½-2 mins until softened. Tip the porridge into bowls and top with the yogurt, banana and seeds.

Cinnamon twists

Ingredients

- 275g whole milk

- 40g unsalted butter, cubed

- 500g strong white flour, plus extra for dusting

- 7g dried active yeast

- 50g caster sugar

- 1 small egg, plus 1 egg, beaten, for glazing

For the filling

- 75g butter, melted

- 150g caster sugar

- 3 tsp ground cinnamon

For the coating

- 50g caster sugar

- 1 tsp ground cinnamon

Instructions

- STEP 1

Heat the milk and butter in a small pan until the butter has melted. Allow to cool slightly – the milk should be warm, not hot. Put the flour in a large mixing bowl with a pinch of salt to one side of the bowl. Add the yeast into the flour on the other side of the bowl, so it's not touching the salt. Pour in the sugar, then mix it all together.

- STEP 2

Gradually pour the warm milk into the dry Ingredients, mixing with your hands until you have a relatively sticky dough. You may not need all of the milk. Add in the egg and continue to work until combined.

• STEP 3

Lightly dust a surface with flour and tip out the dough. It will be quite wet – the more you knead it, the easier it will become. Knead for around 10 mins until you have a smooth dough. Put in a lightly floured bowl to prove for 1 hr or until doubled in size.

• STEP 4

To make the filling, mix the melted butter, sugar and cinnamon together until you get a smooth paste. Set aside.

• STEP 5

Roll out the dough on a lightly floured surface to around a 30 x 40cm rectangle. Spread over the filling using a palette knife until the dough is completely covered.

• STEP 6

Fold in half widthways and cut into 16-18 strips down the shortest side. Twist both ends of each strip in opposite directions until a spiral shape forms. Holding one end in your hand, wrap the rest of the dough around it and over, pressing the ends into the bottom of the bun so it doesn't unravel during cooking.

• STEP 7

Lay on two lined baking trays spaced 5cm apart. Leave to prove for 30-45 mins until risen slightly. Heat the oven to 190C/170C fan/gas 5. Brush the tops of the buns with a little egg and bake for 18-20 mins until golden. Don't worry if a little cinnamon butter comes out.

• STEP 8

For the coating, mix together the sugar and cinnamon. Whilst still warm, toss the buns in the sugar and eat straight away.

Banana & cinnamon pancakes with blueberry compote

Ingredients

- 65g wholemeal flour

- 1 tsp ground cinnamon, plus extra for sprinkling

- 2 egg, plus 2 egg whites

- 100ml whole milk

- 1 small banana, mashed

- ½ tbsp rapeseed oil

- 320g blueberries

- few mint leaves, to serve

Instructions

- STEP 1

Tip the flour and cinnamon into a bowl, then break in the whole eggs, pour in the milk and whisk together until smooth. Stir in the banana. In a separate bowl, whisk the egg whites until light and fluffy, but not completely stiff, then fold into the pancake mix until evenly incorporated.

- STEP 2

Heat a small amount of oil in a large non-stick frying pan, then add a quarter of the pancake mix, swirl to cover the base of the pan and cook until set and golden. Carefully turn the pancake over with a palette knife and cook the other side. Transfer to a plate, then carry on with the rest of the batter until you have four.

- STEP 3

To make the compote, tip the berries in a non-stick pan and heat gently until the berries just burst but hold their shape. Serve two warm pancakes with half the berries, then scatter with the mint leaves and sprinkle with a little cinnamon. Chill the remaining pancakes and compote and serve the next day. You can reheat them in the microwave or in a pan.

Puff pastry cinnamon rolls

Ingredients

- 1½ tbsp ground cinnamon

- 3 tbsp caster sugar

- 320g ready-rolled puff pastry

- plain flour, for dusting

- 1 medium egg, beaten

- 50g icing sugar

Instructions

- STEP 1

Heat the oven to 200C/180C fan/gas 6 and line large baking tray with baking parchment. Stir the cinnamon and sugar together in a small bowl. Unravel the puff pastry on a lightly floured work surface, then sprinkle the cinnamon sugar mixture all over the top. Gently level the cinnamon sugar mixture with the back of a spoon so it covers the pastry almost completely, leaving a 1cm border on one of the short sides. Brush a little of the beaten egg over the exposed pastry border.

- STEP 2

Roll the pastry up in a tight log from the short side without the border. Gently press along the egg-washed border to seal, then slice into 12 equal rounds. Arrange the cinnamon rolls on the prepared baking tray, placing them up against each other so they're just touching. Brush the remaining beaten egg all over the tops and sides of the pastry, then bake for 15-18 mins until golden and risen. Leave to cool on the tray for 10-15 mins.

- STEP 3

Combine the icing sugar with 1½ tsp water in a small bowl until you have a thick icing that easily runs off the spoon. Drizzle this over the warm rolls, then immediately serve.

Salsa verde baked eggs

Ingredients

- 5 tbsp olive oil

- 1 tsp smoked paprika
- 1 tsp cumin seeds
- 400g can cherry tomatoes
- 200g fresh cherry tomatoes
- 2 garlic cloves
- 1 small bunch of parsley
- 1 small bunch of basil
- ½ small bunch of mint, leaves picked
- 2 tbsp capers
- 1 tsp Dijon mustard
- 2 tbsp white wine vinegar
- 200g baby spinach, washed

- 4 eggs

- ½ tsp chilli flakes (optional)

- flatbreads, to serve (optional)

Instructions

- STEP 1

Drizzle 1 tbsp of the olive oil in a frying pan or skillet, and fry the paprika and cumin for 30 seconds over a medium heat. Add the canned tomatoes and fresh tomatoes, bring to the boil, then simmer with a lid on over a medium heat for 5-6 mins until the tomatoes have softened.

- STEP 2

Meanwhile, put the garlic, most of the parsley, the basil, mint, capers, mustard, white wine vinegar, 4 tbsp oil and 3 tbsp cold water in a mini food processor and blitz to a smooth paste. Season.

- STEP 3

Stir the spinach into the pan with the tomatoes until wilted (put the lid back on for a few minutes, then stir again to help it wilt). Make four dips in the mixture and gently crack an egg into each one. Cover with a lid and cook over a medium heat for 6-8 mins, or until the eggs are just set. Uncover the pan, then drizzle over the herby sauce. Scatter over the reserved parsley and chilli flakes, if using. Serve with flatbreads, if you like.

Sweetcorn fritters with eggs & black bean salsa

Ingredients

For the fritters & eggs

- 1 tsp rapeseed oil

- 1 small red onion (85g), finely chopped

- 1 red pepper, deseeded and finely diced

- 100g wholemeal self-raising flour

- 1 tsp smoked paprika

- 1 tsp ground coriander

- 1 tsp baking powder

- 325g can sweetcorn, drained

- 6 large eggs

For the salsa

- 1 small red onion (85g), finely chopped

- 4 tomatoes (320g), chopped

- 2 x 400g cans black beans, drained

- 1 lime, zested and juiced

- ½ x 30g pack coriander, chopped

Instructions

- STEP 1

Heat the oven to 200C/180C fan/gas 6 and line a large baking tray with baking parchment.

- STEP 2

Heat the oil in a small pan and fry the onion and pepper for 5 mins until softened. Meanwhile, mix the flour, spices and baking powder in a bowl. Add the onions, pepper, corn and 2 of the eggs, then mix together well.

- STEP 3

Spoon eight mounds of the mixture onto the baking tray, well-spaced apart, then flatten slightly with the back of the spoon. Bake for 20 mins until set and golden.

- STEP 4

Meanwhile, mix together the salsa Ingredients and poach 2 of the remaining eggs to your liking. Serve the fritters topped with the salsa and the poached eggs.

Nuts & seeds granola

Ingredients

- 150g rolled oats

- 150g mixed nuts (we used whole hazelnuts, flaked almonds and whole pecans)

- 50g mixed seeds (we used a mixed bag containing sunflower, pumpkin, hemp and golden linseed)

- 50g raisins

- 1 tsp ground cinnamon

- ¼ tsp sea salt

- 1 tsp almond extract (vanilla works well too, if you prefer)

- 50ml vegetable oil

- 100ml maple syrup

- milk or yogurt, and fruit (optional), to serve

Instructions

- STEP 1

Heat the oven to 180C/160C fan gas 4. Line a large baking sheet with baking parchment to prevent the granola from sticking. Put all of the dry Ingredients in a large mixing bowl. Whisk together the almond extract, vegetable oil and maple syrup in a jug, then pour into the bowl with the dry Ingredients.

- STEP 2

Mix together well, making sure that all the dry Ingredients are well coated and that there are no dry bits. Tip the mixture onto the lined baking sheet and spread out in an even layer. Cook for about 25-30 mins until golden. You will need to give the mixture a few turns every 8-10 mins to make sure it dries out evenly and doesn't clump together too much. Keep an eye on it as nuts can burn easily.

- STEP 3

Remove from the oven and leave to cool completely on the tray. Break up any large clumps of granola with a wooden spoon. Will keep for up to one month in an airtight container. Serve with milk or yogurt, and fresh seasonal fruit, if you like.

Banana & cinnamon pancakes with blueberry compote

Ingredients

- 65g wholemeal flour

- 1 tsp ground cinnamon, plus extra for sprinkling

- 2 egg, plus 2 egg whites

- 100ml whole milk

- 1 small banana, mashed

- ½ tbsp rapeseed oil

- 320g blueberries

- few mint leaves, to serve

Instructions

- STEP 1

Tip the flour and cinnamon into a bowl, then break in the whole eggs, pour in the milk and whisk together until smooth. Stir in the banana. In a separate bowl, whisk the egg whites until light and fluffy, but not completely stiff, then fold into the pancake mix until evenly incorporated.

- STEP 2

Heat a small amount of oil in a large non-stick frying pan, then add a quarter of the pancake mix, swirl to cover the base of the pan and cook until set and golden.

Carefully turn the pancake over with a palette knife and cook the other side. Transfer to a plate, then carry on with the rest of the batter until you have four.

- STEP 3

To make the compote, tip the berries in a non-stick pan and heat gently until the berries just burst but hold their shape. Serve two warm pancakes with half the berries, then scatter with the mint leaves and sprinkle with a little cinnamon. Chill the remaining pancakes and compote and serve the next day. You can reheat them in the microwave or in a pan.

Almond crêpes with avocado & nectarines

Ingredients

- 2 large eggs

- 3 tbsp ground almonds

- 2 tsp rapeseed oil

- 1 avocado, halved, stoned and flesh lightly crushed

- 2 ripe nectarines, stoned and sliced

- seeds from 1/2 pomegranate

- ½ lime, cut into 2 wedges, for squeezing over

Instructions

- STEP 1

Beat one egg and 1 1 /2 tbsp of the almonds in a small bowl with 1 tbsp water. Heat 1 tsp oil in a large non-stick frying pan over a medium heat and pour in the egg mixture, swirling the pan to evenly cover the base. Cook until the mixture sets and turns golden on the underside, about 2 mins. (There is no need to flip it over.) Turn it out onto a plate and make another one with 1 tbsp water, the remaining egg, oil and almonds.

• STEP 2

Top each crêpe with the avocado, nectarines and pomegranate, and squeeze over the lime at the table.

Millet porridge with almond milk & berry compote

Ingredients

- 340g millet

- 1 litre unsweetened fortified almond milk, plus extra to serve

- few mint leaves, to serve

For the compote

- 90g pitted dates, finely chopped

- 500g frozen mixed fruit (ours was a mixed bag of berries, cherries, currants and strawberries)

- 1 cinnamon stick

Instructions

- STEP 1

For the compote, put the dates in a pan with 150ml water, bring to the boil and stir well so they break down. Tip in the frozen fruit and cinnamon stick and cook over a medium heat, stirring every now and then for a couple of minutes. Don't worry about fully thawing larger fruits, as they will defrost in the residual heat and retain their shape in the compote (if you have large strawberries in the mix, you can halve these as they soften). Leave to cool. Will then keep chilled for up to four days.

- STEP 2

Rinse the millet in a sieve, then tip into a deep, heavy-based saucepan and pour in the almond milk and 350ml water. Put over a low heat and once bubbling, leave to simmer for 10-12 mins, stirring frequently until the millet grains are tender, but nutty.

Serve the porridge with the compote. Add a little extra almond milk to serve with a few mint leaves scattered over.

Berry omelette

Ingredients

- 1 large egg

- 1 tbsp skimmed milk

- 3 pinches of cinnamon

- ½ tsp rapeseed oil

- 100g cottage cheese

- 175g chopped strawberry, blueberries and raspberries

Instructions

- STEP 1

Beat egg with milk and cinnamon. Heat oil in a 20cm non-stick frying pan and pour in the egg mixture, swirling to evenly cover the base. Cook for a few mins until set and golden underneath. There's no need to flip it over.

- STEP 2

Place on a plate, spread over cheese, then scatter with berries. Roll up and serve.

Creamy smoked haddock & saffron kedgeree

Ingredients

- 300g basmati rice

- 50g butter

- 3 hard-boiled eggs, shelled and halved

- 200ml double cream

- 500g naturally smoked haddock, skin removed

- 100ml white wine

- 1tsp cayenne pepper

- pinch saffron strands

- 1 tbsp mild curry powder

- freshly grated nutmeg

- small handful flat-leaf parsley, chopped

- 1 lemon, cut into wedges, to serve

Instructions

- STEP 1

Cook basmati rice, leave to cool. Heat oven to 160C/140C fan/gas 3. Grease a large ovenproof dish with some of the butter. Push the egg yolks through a sieve and roughly chop the whites.

- STEP 2

Gently heat the cream in a frying pan until just below boiling point, then add the fish. Cover and poach for 4 mins. Place the wine in a pan with the saffron and warm to infuse. In a large bowl, mix together the rice, cayenne, curry powder, nutmeg, seasoning, chopped egg whites and saffron-infused wine. Lift the fish out of the cream and flake into the bowl – removing any bones as you find them. Scrape in the cream and gently mix together once more.

• STEP 3

Tip everything into the buttered dish and dot the top with the remaining butter. Bake to heat through for 20 mins, then serve scattered with the parsley and sieved egg yolk, with lemon wedges on the side.

Kale & salmon kedgeree

Ingredients

- 300g brown rice

- 2 salmon fillets (about 280g)

- 4 eggs

- 1 tbsp vegetable oil

- 1 onion, finely chopped

- 100g curly kale, stalks removed, roughly chopped

- 1 garlic clove, crushed

- 1 tbsp curry powder

- 1 tsp turmeric

- zest and juice 1 lemon

Instructions

- STEP 1

Cook the rice following pack instructions. Meanwhile, season the salmon and steam over a pan of simmering water for 8 mins or until just cooked. Keep the pan of water on the heat, add the eggs and boil for 6 mins, then run under cold water.

- STEP 2

Heat the oil in a large frying pan or wok, add the onion and cook for 5 mins. Throw in the kale and cook, stirring, for 5 mins. Add the garlic, curry powder, turmeric and rice, season and stir until heated through.

- STEP 3

Peel and quarter the eggs. Flake the salmon and gently fold through the rice, then divide between plates and top with the eggs. Sprinkle over the lemon zest and squeeze over a little juice before serving.

Cured salmon

Ingredients

- 1 tbsp cracked black pepper

- 75g muscovado sugar

- 60g sea salt flakes

- 1 filleted side of very fresh salmon (about 800g), skin on

For the dill & lemon cream cheese

- 200g full-fat cream cheese, at room temperature

- small bunch of dill, finely chopped

- ½ unwaxed lemon, zested and juiced, plus extra wedges to serve

For the pickle

- 1 small cucumber

- 1 small red onion, finely sliced

- pinch of caster sugar

- 3 tbsp white wine vinegar

To serve

- selection of toasted bagels

- sliced rye bread

- small pot of salmon caviar

- caper berries or capers, drained

Instructions

- STEP 1

Up to four days but at least two days before serving the salmon, mix the pepper, sugar and salt together. Pat the salmon dry with kitchen paper and run your hands over the flesh to find any stray bones – use tweezers to pull these out, if needed. Lay the salmon in a dish, skin-side down, and pack the salt mix over the flesh. Cover the fish with a board or tray weighed down with a few heavy cans or jars. Transfer to the fridge for at least two days or up to four, turning the fillet about every 12 hrs.

- STEP 2

To make the dill cream cheese, beat all of the Ingredients together and set aside. This can be made up to a day ahead and chilled.

- STEP 3

To make the pickle, cut the cucumber in half lengthways, scoop out the seeds using a spoon, and slice into thin half-moons. Toss the cucumber with the red onion and a generous pinch of salt in a colander, then set aside for 30 mins to soften. Transfer the vegetables to a bowl or jar and top up with the sugar and vinegar. Can be eaten immediately or made up to two days ahead and chilled.

- STEP 4

Lift the salmon out of the curing mixture and wipe off any excess seasoning using kitchen paper. Put the fish on a large serving board and carve into thin slices. Serve with the bagels and rye bread, dill & lemon cream cheese, the pickle, salmon caviar, capers and lemon wedges.

SAVORY RECIPES AND MEAL IDEAS FOR LUNCH

Scandi trout with fennel potato salad

Ingredients

- 800g new potatoes

- 1 small red onion, halved and thinly sliced

- 1 small fennel bulb, cored and thinly sliced, fronds reserved

- juice and zest 1 lemon

- 1 tbsp wholegrain mustard

- 1 tsp clear honey

- 1 tbsp olive oil

- 4 trout fillets, skin on

- 100g soured cream

- ½ small pack dill, leaves finely chopped

- ½ small pack flat-leaf parsley, leaves finely chopped

Directions

- STEP 1

Heat oven to 200C/180C fan/gas 6. Put the potatoes in a pan of boiling salted water and simmer for 15 mins until cooked, then drain. Put the onion and fennel in a bowl, cover with the lemon juice and set aside. Mix half the lemon zest with the mustard, honey and oil. Place the trout, skin-side down, on a baking tray lined with parchment. Brush the mustard glaze over the trout and bake in the oven for 10 mins until just cooked and starting to flake.

- STEP 2

Once the potatoes are cool enough to handle, slice them into 1 cm-thick pieces and tip into a large bowl. Mix the remaining lemon zest with the soured cream, dill, parsley and some seasoning. Spoon over the potatoes and stir through. Add the onion and fennel, and mix gently. Sprinkle the reserved fennel fronds over and serve with the trout.

Tuna with peppery tomatoes & potatoes

Ingredients

- 4 tuna steaks

- 1 tbsp olive oil

- 3 garlic cloves, crushed

- few thyme sprigs

- 500g bag new potato, sliced about 1cm thick

- 2 red peppers, cut into large chunks

- 1 red onion, cut into eighths

- 1 green chilli, deseeded and chopped

- 400g can cherry tomato

Directions

- STEP 1

Heat oven to 220C/fan 200C/gas 7 and put in a roasting tin to heat up. Put the tuna in a shallow dish with half the oil, two-thirds of the garlic and leaves from 1 sprig of thyme. Leave to marinate while you cook the veg.

- STEP 2

Put the potatoes, peppers, onion and chilli into the roasting tin with the remaining oil, toss to coat, then roast for 20 mins. The potatoes should be tender or very nearly there. If not, give them another 5 mins (the cooking time can depend on the variety of potato). Add the remaining garlic and thyme to the pan, let them sizzle, stir in the tomatoes, then cook for 5 mins more until the sauce has reduced a little. Season to taste.

- STEP 3

With a few mins to go, heat a griddle or frying pan, wipe most of the garlic marinade off the fish with kitchen paper, season, then sear for 1 min each side for medium or longer if you prefer. Serve on top of the veg.

Fresh salmon with Thai noodle salad

Ingredients

- 2 skinless salmon fillets

- 1 large orange, the juice and zest of half, the rest peeled and chopped

- 125g French beans, trimmed and halved

- 50g mange tout, shredded

- 75g frozen peas

- 75g vermicelli rice noodles

- 2 tsp red curry paste

- 1 tsp fish sauce

- 3 spring onions, finely chopped

- half a pack basil or coriander, chopped

Directions

- STEP 1

Put a pan of water on to boil. Line a steamer with baking parchment, add the salmon fillets and scatter with a little of the orange zest. When the water is boiling, add the beans to the pan, put the salmon in the steamer on top and cook for 5 mins. Take the salmon off, and if it is cooked, set aside but add the peas and mange tout to the pan and cook for 1 min more, or if not quite cooked leave on top for the extra min. Drain the veg, but return the boiling water to the pan, add the noodles and leave to soak for 5 mins.

• STEP 2

Put the curry paste and fish sauce in a salad bowl with the orange juice and a little of the remaining zest and the spring onions. Drain the noodles when they are ready and add to the salad bowl, toss well, then add the chopped orange with the basil or coriander and the cooked vegetables. Tip in the juice from the fish, then toss well and serve in bowls with the salmon on top.

Spice-cured tuna tacos

Ingredients

For the fish

- 400g fresh line-caught tuna

- 3 tbsp olive oil

- 2 limes, zested, 1 juiced

- 1 tbsp cumin seeds

- 1 tbsp coriander seeds

- ½ tsp chilli flakes

For the avocado purée

- 3 ripe avocados, de-stoned and peeled

- 3 tbsp coriander leaves

- 1 tbsp pickle liquor from the pickled jalapeño chillies

To serve

- 8small soft flour tacos

- vegetable oil, for brushing and drizzling

- pickled jalapeño chillies

- 50g pomegranate seeds

- 1bunch coriander, chopped, with a few leaves left whole

- 4 shredded spring onions

- 2 limes, cut into wedges

Directions

- STEP 1

Slice the tuna into 1cm strips, then dice into rough 1cm cubes. Drizzle over the olive oil and scatter over the lime zest, stir and put in the fridge for 20 mins or so. Gently toast the cumin and coriander in a small frying pan, then tip into a pestle and mortar with a pinch of salt and the chilli flakes and crush to a coarse powder. Stir the spice mix into the tuna with the lime juice and put the bowl back in the fridge for at least 10 mins or up to 1 hr.

- STEP 2

To make the avocado purée, put all the Ingredients in a food processor with a pinch of salt and blitz until you have a smooth purée, adding a little oil if it's too thick to blitz. Spoon the mixture into a container.

- STEP 3

If you like your tacos crispy, heat oven to 180C/160C fan/gas 4, brush them with a little oil, place on a baking sheet and cook for 10-15 mins. To build each taco, spoon on some avocado purée and spread out to the edge. Spoon on the spiced tuna and sprinkle over the chillies, pomegranate seeds, coriander and spring onions, drizzle with more oil and add a lime wedge to the plate. Eat with your hands, if soft, or a knife and fork if crispy.

Cheesy seafood bake

Ingredients

- 300g medium potatoes (about 3), thinly sliced

- 2 tbsp milk

- 40g mature cheddar, finely grated

- 1 tsp rapeseed oil

- 1 onion (160g), finely chopped

- 1 red pepper, deseeded and finely diced (270g)

- 2 tsp balsamic vinegar

- 1 tsp vegetable bouillon powder

- 400g can chopped tomatoes

- ½ x 30g pack basil, leaves picked and finely chopped

- 1 garlic clove, finely grated

- 280g pack skinless cod loins

- 100g frozen small Atlantic cooked prawns, defrosted

- 160g broccoli florets

Directions

- STEP 1

Boil the potato slices for 10 mins then drain, tip into a bowl and gently mix in the milk and half the cheese. Don't worry if the potatoes break up a little.

- STEP 2

Meanwhile, heat the oil in a large frying pan and cook the onion until softened. Stir in the pepper and cook for 5 mins more. Spoon in the balsamic vinegar and bouillon powder, then stir in the tomatoes, basil and garlic. Lay the cod fillets on top, then cover and cook for 6-8 mins until the cod flakes when tested. Heat the grill to high.

- STEP 3

Take off the heat, stir in the prawns and tip into a shallow baking dish, breaking up the cod into large chunks. Cover with the potatoes and sprinkle with the remaining cheese. Grill until golden. While it's grilling, steam or boil the broccoli to serve with the bake.

BBQ mackerel

Ingredients

- 3 tbsp extra-virgin olive oil

- 4 small whole mackerel, gutted and cleaned

For the drizzle

- 1 large red chilli, deseeded and finely chopped

- 1 small garlic clove, finely chopped

- small knob fresh root ginger, finely chopped

- 2 tsp honey

- 2 limes, zested and juiced

- 1 tsp sesame oil

- 1 tsp Thai fish sauce

Directions

- STEP 1

Light the barbecue and allow the flames to die down until the ashes have gone white with heat. Make the drizzle by whisking 2 tbsp olive oil and all the other Ingredients together in a small bowl, adjusting the ratio of honey and lime to make a sharp sweetness. Season to taste.

- STEP 2

Score each side of the mackerel about 6 times, not quite through to the bone. Brush the fish with the remaining oil and season lightly. Barbecue the mackerel for 5-6 mins on each side until the fish is charred and the eyes have turned white. Spoon the drizzle over the fish and allow to stand for 2-3 mins before serving.

Korean fishcakes with fried eggs & spicy salsa

Ingredients

For the fishcakes

- 4 x loch trout or rainbow trout fillets, skinned and cut into 1cm/ 1/2in pieces (about 450g/1lb fish)

- 2 tsp finely grated ginger

- 1 fat garlic clove, crushed

- 1 tsp light soy sauce

- bunch spring onions, thinly sliced

- 1 large egg white, beaten until frothy

- 2 tbsp rice flour

- 2 ½ tbsp vegetable oil, for frying

For the salad

- 1 pointed or small white cabbage, cored and finely shredded (about 350g/12oz)

- 100g radishes, thinly sliced

- 2 tbsp Chinese rice vinegar

- 1 tbsp sesame oil, plus 2 tsp to serve

- 1 tsp gochujang, plus 2 top to serve (see tip)

- 1 tsp golden caster sugar

- 1 garlic clove, crushed

- 2 tsp light soy sauce

- 4 medium eggs

- 1 tbsp sesame seeds, toasted

- 1 red chilli, finely sliced, to serve (optional)

Directions

- STEP 1

For the fishcakes, mix the fish with the ginger, garlic, soy and half the spring onions. Stir in the egg white and rice flour.

- STEP 2

Toss the cabbage and radishes with the vinegar, 1 tbsp sesame oil, 1 tsp gochujang, the sugar and garlic. Set aside. Stir together the remaining sesame oil, gochujang and the soy sauce to make a drizzling sauce for later.

- STEP 3

Heat 1 tbsp oil in a large, non-stick frying pan. Split the fish mixture into eight, then spoon four into the pan, pressing the mix to make cakes about 8cm across. Fry for 2 mins each side until just cooked through and golden. Add another 1 tbsp oil to the pan and repeat with the remaining fish. Keep warm in a low oven.

- STEP 4

Add the remaining oil to the pan. Fry the eggs for 2-3 mins until crisp but with a runny yolk. Serve the fishcakes with the cabbage, and top with the egg and sesame seeds. Scatter with the rest of the spring onions, red chilli (if using) and some of the chilli sesame drizzle.

Classic lasagne

Ingredients

- 2 olive oil, plus extra for the dish

- 750g lean beef mince

- 90g pack prosciutto

- 800g passata or half our basic tomato sauce

- 200ml hot beef stock

- nutmeg

- 300g fresh lasagne sheets

- white sauce (find a recipe in the Directions, or use shop-bought)

- 125g ball mozzarella, torn into thin strips

Directions

- STEP 1

To make the meat sauce, heat 2 tbsp olive oil in a frying pan and cook 750g lean beef mince in two batches for about 10 mins until browned all over.

- STEP 2

Finely chop 4 slices of prosciutto from a 90g pack, then stir through the meat mixture.

- STEP 3

Pour over 800g passata or half our basic tomato sauce recipe and 200ml hot beef stock. Add a little grated nutmeg, then season.

- STEP 4

Bring up to the boil, then simmer for 30 mins until the sauce looks rich.

- STEP 5

Heat the oven to 180C/160C fan/gas 4 and lightly oil an ovenproof dish (about 30 x 20cm).

- STEP 6

Spoon one third of the meat sauce into the dish, then cover with some fresh lasagne sheets from a 300g pack. Drizzle over roughly 130g ready-made or homemade white sauce.

- STEP 7

Repeat until you have three layers of pasta. Cover with the remaining 390g white sauce, making sure you can't see any pasta poking through.

- STEP 8

Scatter 125g torn mozzarella over the top.

- STEP 9

Arrange the rest of the prosciutto on top. Bake for 45 mins until the top is bubbling and lightly browned.

Haddock in tomato basil sauce

Ingredients

- 1 tbsp olive oil

- 1 onion, thinly sliced

- 1 small aubergine, about 250g/9oz, roughly chopped

- ½ tsp ground paprika

- 2 garlic cloves, crushed

- 400g can chopped tomato

- 1 tsp dark or light muscovado sugar

- 8 large basil leaves, plus a few extra for sprinkling

- 4 4x175g/6oz firm skinless white fish fillets, such as haddock

Directions

- STEP 1

Heat the olive oil in a large non-stick frying pan and stirfry the onion and aubergine. After about 4 minutes the vegetables will start to turn golden but won't be soft yet, so cover with a lid and let the vegetables steam-fry in their own juices for 6 minutes – this helps them to soften without needing to add any extra oil.

- STEP 2

Stir in the paprika, garlic, tomatoes and sugar with 1/2 tsp salt and cook for another 8-10 minutes, stirring, until onion and aubergine are tender.

- STEP 3

Scatter in the basil leaves then nestle the fish in the sauce, cover the pan and cook for 6-8 minutes until the fish flakes when tested with a knife and the flesh is firm but still moist. Tear over the rest of the basil and serve with a salad and crusty bread.

Antipasti salmon

Ingredients

- 100g sundried tomatoes in oil, drained and finely chopped

- small handful of basil, finely chopped, plus a few whole basil leaves

- small handful of dill, finely chopped, plus a few dill fronds to serve

- 2 tbsp capers, drained and rinsed

- 2 garlic cloves, crushed

- 1 lemon, zested and sliced

- 150g butter, softened

- 600g side of salmon, descaled and pin bones removed

- 3 tbsp pitted black olives

- 100g griddled artichoke hearts, drained and roughly chopped

Directions

- STEP 1

Put the tomatoes, half the herbs, 1 tbsp capers, the garlic, lemon zest and butter in a bowl and mash together with a spoon. Alternatively, tip into a food processor and blitz until combined. The flavoured butter will keep, chilled, for up to two days.

- STEP 2

Layer a sheet of baking parchment large enough to loosely wrap the salmon over an equally-sized sheet of foil. Place the salmon on top, then cut the fish into portions, without cutting all the way through to the skin, so the fillet remains intact. Make the portions as big or small as you like, depending on how many you're feeding. Spread the flavoured butter over the salmon, then top with the remaining capers, the lemon slices, olives and artichokes. Wrap the foil and parchment over the salmon and scrunch the ends to seal, creating a loose parcel.

- STEP 3

To bake the salmon, heat the oven to 200C/180C fan/gas 6. Put the parcel on a baking tray and cook for 30 mins, then leave to stand for a few minutes before unwrapping. Alternatively, light the barbecue, wait for the flames to die down, put the parcel directly on the grill and cook for 8-15 mins, or until the salmon is cooked through. Check the salmon is cooked by pushing the flesh with a fork – it should easily flake. Serve on a platter, scattered with the remaining herbs and the buttery juices poured over.

Sticky onion & cheddar quiche

Ingredients

- 25g butter

- 500g small onion, (about 5 in total), halved and finely sliced

- 2 eggs

- 284ml pot double cream

- 140g mature cheddar, coarsely grated

For the pastry

- 280g plain flour, plus extra for dusting

- 140g cold butter

Directions

- STEP 1

To make the pastry, tip the flour and butter into a bowl, then rub together with your fingertips until completely mixed and crumbly. Add 8 tbsp cold water, then bring everything together with your hands until just combined. Roll into a ball and use straight away or chill for up to 2 days. The pastry can also be frozen for up to a month.

- STEP 2

Roll out the pastry on a lightly floured surface to a round about 5cm larger than a 25cm tin. Use your rolling pin to lift it up, then drape over the tart case so there is an overhang of pastry on the sides. Using a small ball of pastry scraps, push the pastry into the corners of the tin (see picture, above left). Chill in the fridge or freezer for 20 mins.

- STEP 3

Heat oven to 200C/fan 180C/gas 6. While the pastry is chilling, heat the butter in a pan and cook the onions for 20 mins, stirring occasionally, until they become sticky and golden. Remove from the heat.

- STEP 4

Lightly prick the base of the tart with a fork, line the tart case with a large circle of greaseproof paper or foil, then fill with baking beans. Blind-bake the tart for 20 mins, remove the paper and beans, then continue to cook for 5-10 mins until biscuit brown.

- STEP 5

Meanwhile, beat the eggs in a bowl, then gradually add the cream. Stir in the onions and half the cheese, then season with salt and pepper. Carefully tip the filling into the case, sprinkle with the rest of the cheese, then bake for 20-25 mins until set and golden. Leave to cool in the case, trim the edges of the pastry, then remove and serve in slices.

Steamed bass with pak choi

Ingredients

- small piece of ginger, peeled and sliced

- 2 garlic cloves, finely sliced

- 3 spring onions, finely sliced

- 2 tbsp soy sauce

- 1 tbsp sesame oil

- splash of sherry (optional)

- 2 x fillets sea bass

- 2 heads pak choi, quartered

Directions

- STEP 1

In a small bowl, mix all of the Ingredients, except the fish and the pak choi, together to make a soy mix. Line one tier of a two-tiered bamboo steamer loosely with foil. Lay the fish, skin side up, on the foil and spoon over the soy mix. Place the fish over simmering water and throw the pak choi into the second tier and cover it with a lid. Alternatively, add the pak choi to the fish layer after 2 mins of cooking – the closer the tier is to the steam, the hotter it is.

- STEP 2

Leave everything to steam for 6-8 mins until the pak choi has wilted and the fish is cooked. Divide the greens between two plates, then carefully lift out the fish. Lift the foil up and drizzle the tasty juices back over the fish.

Mackerel with orange & harissa glaze

Ingredients

- 2 x 300g/10oz mackerel, filleted and skin on or 4 x 75g/3oz mackerel fillets, skin on

- 2 tbsp plain flour

- ½ tsp smoked paprika

- 2 tbsp extra-virgin olive oil

- 1small orange, grated zest and juice

- 1-2 tsp harissa paste (to taste, as brands vary)

- 50g pine nut, toasted

- small bunch coriander, very roughly chopped

Directions

- STEP 1

Roll the mackerel fillets in the flour sifted with smoked paprika and seasoning. Shake off excess flour and set the fish aside in a single layer.

- STEP 2

Put 1 tbsp of the olive oil, the orange zest and juice and the harissa paste into a small bowl, and whisk together. Heat a frying pan with remaining olive oil until very hot. Fry the fish fillets for 5 mins, first on the skin side, then on the flesh side.

• STEP 3

When the fish is nearly cooked – it should look firm – pour over the orange and harissa glaze, bring to the boil and allow the liquid to bubble until sticky. Sprinkle over the pine nuts and coriander.

Wild salmon with coconut chutney & green pilau

Ingredients

- 1 tsp rapeseed oil

- 1 onion, sliced

- 25g ginger, cut into thin matchsticks

- 2 garlic cloves, chopped

- 1 green chilli, deseeded and sliced

- ⅔ small pack coriander

- handful mint leaves

- 20g creamed coconut

- 1 lime, zested and 1/2 juiced

- 50g brown basmati rice

- 2 x 100g skinless wild salmon fillets, thawed if frozen

- head of spring greens (about 175g), stalks trimmed, finely shredded (remove outer leaves if tough)

- 125g frozen peas

- 1 tbsp ground coriander

Directions

- STEP 1

Heat oven to 200C/180C fan/ gas 6. Heat the oil in a large non-stick wok and add the onion, ginger, garlic and chilli. Cook briefly over a high heat to mix everything, then cover and leave to cook gently for about 10 mins until the onions are soft. Scoop two spoonfuls of the mixture into a bowl, add the coriander, mint, coconut, lime zest and juice with 1 tbsp water and blitz to a purée with a stick bender.

- STEP 2

Meanwhile, boil the rice for 20 mins, then drain.

- STEP 3

Spread half the coconut mixture over the fish and wrap up in a parcel of foil. Bake for 10 mins.

- STEP 4

Carry on cooking the onions, uncovered this time, until they start to brown. Add the spring greens and stir-fry for a few mins until softened. Add the rice and peas with the ground coriander and cook until the veg is tender. If the mixture starts to stick, add 1 tbsp water. Stir through the remaining coconut mixture, then serve with the fish.

SAVORY RECIPES AND MEAL IDEAS FOR DINNER

Tomato & thyme cod

Ingredients

- 1 tbsp olive oil

- 1 onion, chopped

- 400g can chopped tomatoes

- 1 heaped tsp light soft brown sugar

- few sprigs thyme, leaves stripped

- 1 tbsp soy sauce

- 4 cod fillets, or another white flaky fish, such as pollock

Directions

- STEP 1

Heat 1 tbsp olive oil in a frying pan, add 1 chopped onion, then fry for 5-8 mins until lightly browned.

- STEP 2

Stir in a 400g can chopped tomatoes, 1 heaped tsp light soft brown sugar, the leaves from a few sprigs of thyme and 1 tbsp soy sauce, then bring to the boil.

- STEP 3

Simmer 5 mins, then slip 4 cod fillets into the sauce.

- STEP 4

Cover and gently cook for 8-10 mins until the cod flakes easily. Serve with baked or steamed potatoes.

Creamy salmon, leek & potato traybake

Ingredients

- 250g baby potatoes, thickly sliced

- 2 tbsp olive oil

- 1 leek, halved, washed and sliced

- 1 garlic clove, crushed

- 70ml double cream

- 1 tbsp capers, plus extra to serve

- 1 tbsp chives, plus extra to serve

- 2 skinless salmon fillets

- mixed rocket salad, to serve (optional)

Directions

- STEP 1

Heat the oven to 200C/180C fan/gas 6. Bring a medium pan of water to the boil. Add the potatoes and cook for 8 mins. Drain and leave to steam-dry in a colander for a few minutes. Toss the potatoes with ½ of the oil and plenty of seasoning in a baking tray. Put in the oven for 20 mins, tossing halfway through the cooking time.

- STEP 2

Meanwhile, heat the remaining oil in a frying pan over a medium heat. Add the leek and fry for 5 mins, or until beginning to soften. Stir through the garlic for 1 min, then add the cream, capers and 75ml hot water, then bring to the boil. Stir through the chives.

- STEP 3

Heat the grill to high. Pour the creamy leek mixture over the potatoes, then sit the salmon fillets on top.

Grill for 7-8 mins, or until just cooked through. Serve topped with extra chives and capers and a salad on the side, if you like.

Crushed new potato fish cakes with horseradish mayonnaise

Ingredients

- 750g new potato, cut into large chunks

- 100g baby spinach

- 2 smoked haddock fillets, about 600g

- 700ml whole milk

- 2 bay leaves

- ½ tsp black peppercorns

- 1 egg yolk

- 2 tbsp vegetable oil

- 25g plain flour

- lemon wedges, to serve

For the horseradish mayo

- 250ml mayonnaise

- 50g fresh horseradish, grated (or from a jar)

- juice and zest ½ lemon

Directions

- STEP 1

Cook the potatoes in boiling salted water for 10-15 mins until tender. Drain in a colander over the spinach so the leaves wilt. Return the potatoes to the pan to steam-dry, then roughly crush with a fork. Leave to cool.

- STEP 2

In a separate pan, poach the haddock in the milk with the bay leaves and peppercorns for 4 mins. Turn off the heat and leave to cook for a few mins more until the flesh flakes. Remove to a plate and break into large pieces, discarding the skin and any bones.

- STEP 3

Mix the cooled potato, wilted spinach and haddock with the egg yolk and 3 tbsp of the poaching milk. Form into 4 chunky cakes and chill in the fridge, covered, for at least 30 mins, or overnight. Mix all the mayonnaise Ingredients together and chill.

- STEP 4

Heat the oil in a large pan over a medium heat. Sprinkle flour over the fish cakes and fry for about 5-6 mins on each side until golden and heated through.

Serve with lemon wedges and a dollop of the horseradish mayo.

Spicy Singaporean fish

Ingredients

- 2 red chillies, deseeded and chopped

- 2 shallots, chopped

- 1 garlic clove, chopped

- 1 lemongrass, outer leaves removed, chopped

- small knob ginger peeled and chopped

- 2 tsp soy sauce

- pinch sugar

- 2 tbsp vegetable oil

- 2 fillets lemon sole, about 120g each

- chives and coriander, to serve

Directions

- STEP 1

Make a paste by blending together the chillies, shallots, garlic, lemongrass, ginger, soy sauce and sugar in a blender or coffee grinder, or use a pestle and mortar. Heat the oil in a small frying pan and cook the paste for 2 mins until it has darkened slightly and you can really smell the spices. Season with a little salt if you like, then set aside.

- STEP 2

Heat the grill to medium. Put the fish onto a grill pan, then use the back of a teaspoon to smear the paste all over, making a thin layer covering the whole fish. Pop under the grill and cook for 10 mins until the fish flakes easily. Serve with rice and steamed bok choy. Sprinkle chives and coriander on the fish to serve, if you like.

Spiced fish & mussel pie

Ingredients

- 750g parsnip, peeled, cored and cut into large chunks

- 500g potatoes, peeled and cut into medium-sized chunks

- 85g butter

- 300ml fresh fish stock

- 1kg fresh mussel, scrubbed clean

- 1 large onion, chopped

- 1 tbsp medium curry powder or paste

- 50g plain flour

- 400ml can coconut milk

- 750g Icelandic cod fillet, skinned and cut into large cubes

- 100g cooked tiger prawns

- 1 pack fresh coriander, chopped

Directions

- STEP 1

Boil the parsnips and potatoes for 15-20 mins until tender. Drain and mash well with 25g/1oz butter and seasoning. Cover and set aside.

- STEP 2

Bring the stock to the boil in a large pan. Tip in the mussels, cover and leave to steam for about 3 mins, or until the shells open. Drain into a colander set over a large bowl to reserve the stock. Remove and throw away the shells and any un-opened mussels. Cover the cooked mussels to stop them drying out.

- STEP 3

Melt the remaining butter and fry the onion until softened. Stir in the curry powder and fl our, and cook for about 1 min. Pour in the coconut milk and 3-4 tbsp of the reserved mussel stock and stir well until you have a smooth sauce. Leave to simmer for 5 mins until thickened.

- STEP 4

Add the cod to the sauce, return to a simmer and cook for 3-4 mins, stirring occasionally, but trying not to break up the cod. Stir in the mussels, prawns and coriander, season, then tip into a large ovenproof dish. Spread the parsnip mash over the top.

- STEP 5

To serve now heat the grill and grill until the mash is golden and crusty. To eat later cool, cover, then chill for a couple of hours. To serve, heat oven to 200C/ fan 180C/gas 6 and bake for 35-40 mins until hot all the way through.

Spicy fish cakes with mango dipping sauce

Ingredients

- 1kg medium-sized floury potato such as Maris Piper, unpeeled

- 10 tbsp vegetable oil

- 2 tsp mustard seed

- 2 tbsp curry leaf, fresh or dried

- 2 red onions, finely chopped

- 2 red chillies, deseeded and chopped

- 50g ginger, finely chopped

- zest 1 lemon

- 2 eggs, lightly beaten

- 600g skinless salmon fillet

- 250g skinless smoked haddock

- 300ml milk

For the coating

- 6 tbsp plain flour, seasoned

- 3 eggs, lightly beaten

- 200g fresh white breadcrumb

For the mango dipping sauce

- 4 tbsp mango chutney

- juice 2 limes

- 2 tbsp shredded mint

Directions

- STEP 1

Put the potatoes in a large saucepan, cover with salted water, bring to the boil and cook until tender. Drain, leave to cool, then peel and mash.

- STEP 2

Heat 4 tbsp of the oil in a pan set over a medium heat. Add the mustard seeds, half the curry leaves, onions, red chillies and ginger, and fry for 5 mins until the onions have softened. Add onion mixture to the mashed potato with the lemon zest, mix well, then work in the eggs.

• STEP 3

Put the salmon and smoked haddock in a pan. Add the remaining curry leaves, then pour over the milk plus enough water to cover. Put on the lid and simmer for 3-4 mins, then turn off the heat and leave the fish in the pan for 10 mins to finish cooking. Take the fish out of the milk and leave to cool. Using your hands, break into big flakes, add to the potato mixture and mix gently to combine.

• STEP 4

Shape mixture into patties about 9cm diameter and 3cm thick. For the coating, dust each with flour, then dip into the egg and coat with breadcrumbs. Transfer to a tray lined with baking parchment and chill for 30 mins. The fish cakes can be frozen at this point. Put the tray in the freezer and when frozen, pop the fish cakes in bags and seal.

- STEP 5

Heat the remaining oil in a frying pan and cook the fish cakes, in batches, for 7-8 mins each side, until golden and crisp. Drain on kitchen paper. To cook fish cakes from frozen, see below.

- STEP 6

Combine all the dipping sauce Ingredients and stir in 4-5 tbsp water to thin it down. Serve with the fish cakes.

One-pan Thai green salmon

Ingredients

- 2 tbsp vegetable oil

- 2 shallots, thickly sliced

- 1 green chilli, deseeded if you like, and sliced, plus extra to serve

- 300g baby new potatoes, quartered

- 1 lemongrass stalk, bashed

- 4 tbsp Thai green curry paste

- 400g can coconut milk

- 200-300ml vegetable stock

- 1-2 tbsp fish sauce

- ½-1 tbsp brown or palm sugar

- 1 courgette, trimmed and peeled into ribbons

- 100g baby spinach

- 4 skinless salmon fillets

- 3 limes, 2 juiced plus 1 cut into wedges to serve

- 3 spring onions, finely sliced (optional)

- handful of coriander or Thai basil, roughly chopped, to serve

- cooked jasmine rice or rice noodles, to serve (optional)

Directions

- STEP 1

Heat the oven to 200C/180C fan/ gas 6. Put the oil in a deep roasting tin or dish about 30 x 25cm and toss through the shallots, chilli, potatoes and lemongrass. Roast for 10 mins until fragrant, keeping an eye on the shallots to ensure they don't burn. Remove from the oven and stir in the curry paste to coat everything. Return to the oven for 2 mins until its aroma is released before mixing in the coconut milk and 200ml stock. Put back in the oven again for 15-20 mins until the sauce is slightly thickened and the potatoes are turning tender.

- STEP 2

Season to taste with the fish sauce and sugar, then stir through the courgette ribbons and spinach. Add another 50ml-100ml stock now if the sauce is too thick, but be aware that the courgette and spinach will release some water as well. Nestle the salmon fillets in the sauce and bake for a further 10-15 mins until the salmon is cooked to your liking.

- STEP 3

Add the lime juice and taste the sauce for a balance of sweet and sour, adding more lime juice and fish sauce, if you like. Scatter over the spring onions, if using, along with the herbs and chilli. For a more filling meal, serve with rice or noodles and the lime wedges on the side.

Indian-spiced fish cakes

Ingredients

- 600g potato, quartered if large

- ½ tsp cumin seeds

- 2 spring onions, finely chopped

- 1 red chilli, deseeded and finely chopped

- 2 tbsp chopped coriander

- 1 egg, beaten

- 100g cooked leftover salmon, flaked into large pieces

- plain flour, for coating

- 25g butter and 1 tbsp sunflower oil

- leftover avocado mayo, raita or mango chutney, to serve

Directions

- STEP 1

Boil the potatoes. Meanwhile, dry-fry the cumin seeds for a couple of secs in a large non-stick frying pan. When soft, drain the potatoes, return to the saucepan, add the cumin, onions, chilli and coriander with plenty of seasoning, then mash well. When cooled a little, beat in 2 tbsp of the egg, then carefully stir through the salmon. Shape into 4 rough cakes, then coat in flour. If freezing, freeze on a baking sheet until solid, then pack up.

- STEP 2

In the frying pan, melt the butter with the oil. Fry the cakes for about 2 mins each side until golden. Serve with the mayo, raita (recipe below) or mango chutney and some salad leaves.

Tomato & mascarpone risotto

Ingredients

- 2 tbsp olive oil

- 1 onion, very finely chopped

- 1 large garlic clove, crushed

- 175g risotto rice

- 400g can cherry tomatoes

- 600ml hot vegetable stock

- 30g parmesan or vegetarian alternative, grated

- 30g mascarpone, or cream cheese

- ½ small bunch of basil, chopped

Directions

- STEP 1

Heat the oil in a large, heavy-based saucepan. Add the onion along with a pinch of salt, and fry for 10 mins or until beginning to soften and turn translucent, then add the garlic and fry for 1 min. Stir in the rice and cook for 2 mins.

- STEP 2

Tip in the tomatoes and bring to a simmer. Add half the stock, cooking and stirring until absorbed. Add the remaining stock, a ladleful at a time, and cook until the rice is al dente, stirring constantly for around 20 mins.

- STEP 3

Stir through the parmesan, mascarpone or cream cheese, and basil, then season to taste. Spoon into bowls to serve.

Mustard salmon & veg bake with horseradish sauce

Ingredients

- 4 parsnips, sliced lengthways

- 4 small raw beetroot, thickly sliced

- 6 carrots, sliced lengthways

- 2 tbsp olive oil

- 4 x 125g/4½oz pieces salmon with skin

- 2 tbsp grainy mustard

- 2 tbsp hot horseradish

- 150ml crème fraîche

- 1 tbsp cider vinegar

- 1 tbsp chopped dill

Directions

- STEP 1

Heat oven to 200C/180C fan/gas 6. Toss all the vegetables with the oil and season well. Spread in a single layer on 2 baking trays (or 1 very large tray) and roast for 30 mins.

- STEP 2

Season the salmon and spread over the mustard. In the final 10 mins of cooking the veg, add the salmon to the trays.

- STEP 3

In a small bowl, mix together the horseradish, crème fraîche, vinegar, dill and some seasoning. Serve the salmon with the sauce and veg.

Hake fish cakes with mustard middles

Ingredients

For the fish cakes

- 450g floury potatoes, cut into chunks (we used Rooster potatoes)

- 1 bay leaf

- a few peppercorns

- 450g skinless hake fillet, cut into 4

- bunch spring onions, finely shredded

- 1 whole nutmeg

- 3 tbsp plain flour, seasoned

- 1 egg

- 100g fresh breadcrumbs

- 2l vegetable oil, for deep-frying

- salad leaves, to serve

- lemon wedges, to serve

For the mustard middles

- 100g full-fat crème fraîche

- 50g strong cheddar, grated

- 1 egg yolk (reserve the white)

- 1 tbsp wholegrain mustard

Directions

- STEP 1

Mix all the mustard middle Ingredients together. Drape cling film across a muffin tin, then spoon the mix into 4 of the wells. Freeze for 30 mins or until solid.

- STEP 2

Put the potatoes, bay leaf and peppercorns in a pan of cold water, bring to the boil and cook for 20 mins or until tender. Remove and allow to steam-dry in a colander. Add the fish to the water and simmer for 5 mins until it is just cooked through at the thickest part.

- STEP 3

Mash the potatoes and stir in the spring onions, a little freshly grated nutmeg and some seasoning. Drain the hake, then flake it into the mash. Gently mix everything together and leave to cool.

- STEP 4

Divide the fish mixture into 4. Shape 1 fish cake at a time, moulding it into a ball. Make a well in the centre of the ball and push a frozen mustard middle into it, then shape the mash around it to make a smooth hockey-puck shape. Repeat with the remaining fish, then freeze for 15 mins.

- STEP 5

Using 3 shallow bowls, add the flour to one; put the egg and reserved egg white in another, and the breadcrumbs in the third. Beat the eggs with some seasoning. Thoroughly coat the fishcakes first in the flour, then the egg , then the breadcrumbs. Freeze the fish cakes until firm. Can be frozen for up to 1 month – defrost in the fridge for 2 hrs before cooking.

- STEP 6

When ready to cook, heat the oil to 180C in a large, deep saucepan (or use a fat fryer) and the oven to

190C/170C fan/gas 5. Fry the fish cakes for 7 mins, turning halfway, until crisp. Drain on kitchen paper, transfer to a baking sheet and bake for 5 mins (15 mins from frozen) so the middles are hot. Serve with dressed leaves and a lemon wedge.

Baked sea bream with tomatoes & coriander

Ingredients

- 4 large potatoes, about 1kg/2lb 4oz

- 2 garlic cloves, finely chopped

- pinch dried chilli flakes

- pinch saffron

- 1 bunch coriander, roughly chopped

- 4 whole sea bream, cleaned and gutted

- 1 tbsp olive oil, plus extra for greasing

- juice 2 limes

- 125ml white wine

- handful sundried tomatoes

- handful pine nuts, toasted

- 4 thin slices pancetta or smoked streaky bacon

Directions

- STEP 1

Heat the oven to 200C/180C fan/gas 6. Slice the potatoes thinly, put in a large saucepan and cover with cold salted water. Bring to the boil and drain, then lay onto the base of a lightly oiled large baking tray. Scatter over the garlic, chilli, saffron and a little of the coriander.

• STEP 2

Slash the fish through the flesh down to the bone – this allows it to cook evenly and quicker than normal. Season and rub with the olive oil. Lay the fish on the potatoes and top with the lime juice, wine, tomatoes and pine nuts. Lay the pancetta slices over the fish and bake for 20-25 mins or until the fish is cooked through. Check by pulling out one of the fins on the back, it should come away easily. Serve the fish scattered with the remaining coriander.

Herby fish fingers

Ingredients

- 50g crustless stale white bread

- finely grated zest of a large lemon

- 2 tbsp each roughly chopped fresh dill, fresh chives and fresh parsley

- 500g skinless lemon sole fillets

- 2 tbsp seasoned flour

- 1 egg, beaten

- vegetable oil, for shallow frying

Directions

- STEP 1

Pulse the bread to coarse crumbs in the food processor. Add the lemon zest, herbs and a pinch of salt, and pulse to make bright green, fine breadcrumbs.

- STEP 2

Cut the lemon sole into thick strips, about 3 x 10cm. Dust each fish piece with the fl our, shake off any excess, then dip into the egg then the breadcrumbs. At this stage, they can be cooked straight away, kept in the fridge for a few hours, or frozen.

- STEP 3

To serve, heat about 1cm of oil in a large frying pan. Once it's nice and hot, fry the fish fingers a few at a time for 1-2 mins on each side. Drain on kitchen paper, and keep warm while you continue with the rest. When they are all cooked, serve straight away with the oven-roasted chips and tartare sauce.

Salmon & lemon mini fish cakes

Ingredients

- 2 large baking potatoes

- 2 tbsp olive oil

- grated zest and juice ½ lemon

- 1 egg yolk

- 140g smoked salmon trimmings, plus extra to serve

- 1 tbsp chopped parsley, plust extra

- 2 tbsp gluten-free flour mixed with 1 tsp coarsely ground pepper

- a little oil, for frying

Directions

- STEP 1

Microwave potatoes on high for 10 mins until tender. Leave to cool for 5 mins, scoop the flesh in a bowl, then mash and leave to cool. Season with olive oil, lemon zest and juice to taste, then mix in the egg, salmon and parsley. Shape into small rounds 3cm wide and 1cm deep. Chill for 15 mins.

- STEP 2

Dust each cake with the peppered flour, then fry over a low heat in a little oil for 2-3 mins on each side. Drain on kitchen paper and serve garnished with salmon and parsley.

SIDE DISH

Cheesy roasted courgettes

Ingredients

- 4 courgettes, halved lengthways

- 250g tub ricotta

- zest 1 lemon

- 1 chilli, deseeded and finely chopped

- handful chopped herbs, such as mint, parsley and basil

- 4 tbsp dried breadcrumbs

Directions

- STEP 1

Heat oven to 200C/180C fan/gas 6. Use a teaspoon to scoop the seeds from the middle of each courgette half, then place them in a large baking tray.

- STEP 2

Mix together the ricotta, zest, chilli and herbs, and season with salt and pepper. Pile the stuffing into the courgettes and top with breadcrumbs. Bake for 35 mins until the courgettes are tender and the topping is golden and crisp.

Baked feta with sesame & honey

Ingredients

- 1 tbsp sesame seeds, toasted

- 200g block feta

- 2 tbsp honey, plus extra to serve

- 1 tsp roughly chopped oregano

- olive oil, for drizzling

- warmed pitta breads, to serve

Directions

- STEP 1

Heat the oven to 200C/180C fan/gas 6, or if using an air-fryer, heat to 180C for 3 mins. Put the sesame seeds in a shallow dish and brush the block of feta all over with the honey. Carefully press the honey-coated feta into the sesame seeds, turning so that it's well crusted with seeds.

- STEP 2

Put the feta in a baking dish (it should fit snugly), then sprinkle over the oregano and a pinch of sea salt. Drizzle with some olive oil. Bake in the oven for 15-20 mins, or cook in the air-fryer for 15 mins until the feta is soft, then drizzle with a little extra honey and serve with the pitta breads on the side.

Smoked haddock & cheddar fishcakes with watercress sauce

Ingredients

- 425g floury potatoes, cut into large chunks

- 1 bay leaf

- 6 peppercorns

- small bunch flat-leaf parsley, leaves and stalks separated

- 225g smoked haddock fillets, skin on (we used dyed haddock to give the mash a lovely golden colour)

- 200g unsmoked haddock fillets, skin on

- 75g mature British cheddar, grated

- 4 spring onions, 0.5 very finely sliced, 0.5 roughly chopped

- 50g plain flour

- 2 medium eggs, beaten

- 100g fresh breadcrumbs

- sunflower oil, for frying

- 50g watercress (weighed after discarding the thickest stalks)

- 4 tbsp rapeseed oil

- 2 lemons, 1 juiced, 1 cut into small wedges to serve (optional)

Directions

- STEP 1

Put the potatoes, bay leaf, peppercorns and parsley stalks in a big pan of cold water. Cover with a lid, bring to the boil and cook for 15 mins until tender. Using a slotted spoon, transfer the potatoes to a colander and leave to steam-dry. Turn the heat down, add the fish and poach gently for 5 mins until it flakes easily. Tip the potatoes into a big bowl and put the fish in the colander to drain for a few mins.

- STEP 2

Add the cheese, some pepper and a little salt to the potatoes and mash well. Flake in about half the fish, discarding the skin and bones, and mash in too. Flake in the remaining fish in big chunks, scatter over the sliced spring onions and gently mix together. Roll the mixture into golf-ball-sized cakes.

- STEP 3

Tip the flour onto a plate and season. Tip the egg and breadcrumbs into 2 shallow bowls each. Roll each fishcake first in the flour, then the egg, then the breadcrumbs. Sit on some parchment-lined trays that fit in your fridge. Chill for at least 1 hr or up to 24 hrs.

- STEP 4

Fill a deep frying pan with 1-2cm of sunflower oil, heat until shimmering, then brown a few fishcakes at a time, turning regularly. If the oil gets too crumby, change halfway through. You can serve them straight away, or cool and chill for up to 24 hrs in the fridge, then simply warm for 30 mins in an oven at 180C/160C fan/ gas 4 before the party.

- STEP 5

Make the dipping sauce up to 1 hr before serving – put the roughly chopped spring onions, the parsley leaves, watercress, rapeseed oil, 2 tbsp lemon juice and 5 tbsp water in a food processor or blender. Whizz to the consistency of single cream.

- STEP 6

Pile the warm fishcakes onto a platter with a bowl of watercress sauce on the side and some lemon wedges for squeezing over, if you like.

Lemon & coriander couscous

Ingredients

- 250g couscous

- grated zest of a lemon

- 2 x 20g packs fresh coriander

- 4 tbsp raisins

- 4 tbsp toasted pine nuts

Directions

- STEP 1

Prepare 250g couscous with boiling water or stock, according to the packet's instructions.

- STEP 2

Add the lemon zest, fresh coriander, raisins and pine nuts. Season well and drizzle with plenty of olive oil. Goes really well with fish or lamb.

Perfect roast potatoes

Ingredients

- 16 potatoes the best ones to use are Desirée, as they hold their shape, but King Edward and Maris Piper are also good

- 2 tbsp plain flour

- 140g goose fat or duck fat or dripping

- 3 tbsp sunflower oil or vegetable oil

Directions

- STEP 1

Heat oven to 190C/fan 170C/gas 5. Peel the potatoes and cut in half; if very large, cut into quarters, or leave whole if they are small. Tip into a saucepan, cover with cold water, then bring to the boil. Set the timer and boil for exactly 2 mins. Drain the potatoes well, then toss in the colander to fluff up their surfaces, sprinkling over the flour as you go.

- STEP 2

Place a large, sturdy roasting tray over a fairly high heat, then tip in the fat and oil. When sizzling, lower in the potatoes carefully, then gently brown in the hot fat for about 5 mins so all the sides are covered with oil.

- STEP 3

Roast undisturbed for 20 mins, then remove from the oven and gently turn them over with a fish slice. Place the tray on the hob to heat the oil, then return to the oven and cook for another 20 mins. Turn again, putting the tray back on the hob to heat the oil. Give them a final 20 mins in the oven, by which time you should have perfect roast potatoes.

Courgette & anchovy salad

Ingredients

- ¼ tsp fennel seed

- juice and zest ½ lemon

- 1 tbsp extra-virgin olive oil, plus extra for drizzling

- 1 garlic clove, crushed

- 1 large courgette, thinly sliced on the diagonal

- 50g rocket

- 2 anchovy fillets, halved

Directions

- STEP 1

Toast the fennel seeds in a small frying pan over a low-medium heat for 1 min, or until they release their aroma. Bash them lightly using a pestle and mortar. Mix the lemon juice, fennel seeds, oil and garlic in a large bowl, then stir in the courgette. Season and set aside to marinate for 30 mins.

• STEP 2

Toss through the rocket and transfer to a platter. Top with the anchovy fillets. Scatter with lemon zest and serve with an extra drizzle of olive oil.

Barbecued fennel with black olive dressing

Ingredients

- 2 fennel bulbs, sliced lengthways into 1cm-thick pieces

- 1 ½ tbsp olive oil

- 2 tbsp finely chopped black Kalamata olive

- 1 garlic clove, crushed

- juice 1 lemon

- small handful each parsley and basil, finely chopped

Directions

- STEP 1

Heat a BBQ or griddle pan. Toss the fennel in 1 tbsp of the oil, coating well. Cook for 5 mins on each side until golden brown and charred.

- STEP 2

To make the dressing, put the olives, garlic, lemon juice and remaining oil in a bowl. Add the chopped herbs and combine. Lay the fennel on a platter and pour over the dressing. Eat warm or at room temperature.

Apricot pancakes with honey butter

Ingredients

For the butter

- 100g butter, softened

- 2 tbsp clear honey

For the pancakes

- 140g self-raising flour

- pinch bicarbonate of soda

- 25g caster sugar

- 1 egg

- 150ml milk

- handful ready-to-eat dried apricots, finely chopped

- oil, for frying

Directions

- STEP 1

For the honey butter, beat the butter with the honey and spoon onto a large piece of cling film. Squeeze into a sausage shape, then wrap tightly and chill until ready to use. Will keep in the fridge for up to a month.

- STEP 2

Sift the flour, bicarbonate of soda and a small pinch of salt into a bowl, then stir through the sugar and make a well in the centre. Beat together the egg and milk, then gradually pour into the well, stirring slowly, to avoid creating lumps. Stir in the apricots.

- STEP 3

Heat a non-stick frying pan over a low heat and add a little oil. Drop in 4 tablespoonfuls of batter and cook for 1 min or until the surface of each pancake is covered in bubbles. Flip with a palette knife or fish slice, then cook for a further min. Repeat with the remaining batter. Serve warm or leave to cool, then toast and spread with the honey butter to serve

Harissa cauliflower pilaf

Ingredients

- 300g basmati rice

- 1 red onion, finely sliced

- 2 lemons, 1 juiced, 1 cut into wedges

- 2 tsp sugar

- 4 tbsp harissa

- 1 garlic clove, crushed

- 1 tbsp olive oil

- 1 large or 2 medium cauliflower, broken into large florets, stalk chopped, large leaves roughly chopped

- pinch of saffron

- 2 bay leaves

- 700ml hot vegan vegetable stock

- 100g sultanas

- 100g flaked almonds, toasted until golden brown

- ½ small bunch of dill, chopped, plus extra to serve

- 400g can chickpeas, drained and rinsed

- 50g pomegranate seeds (optional)

Directions

- STEP 1

Wash the rice really well, then leave to soak in cold water for 1 hr. Put the onion in a small bowl and toss with the lemon juice, the sugar and a pinch of salt. Leave to pickle while you make the pilaf.

- STEP 2

Heat the oven to 200C/180C fan/gas 6. Whisk 2 tbsp harissa, the garlic and oil in a large bowl, then add the cauliflower and toss to coat in the sauce. Season, then tip into a roasting tin and roast for 30 mins until tender and golden.

- STEP 3

Meanwhile, mix the saffron, bay leaves, stock and 2 tbsp harissa in a pan over a very low heat to keep warm while the cauli roasts.

- STEP 4

Remove the cauli from the oven, tip into a dish and squeeze over the juice from one of the lemon wedges. Drain the rice and tip into the roasting tin. Pour over the infused stock, and mix well. Stir in the sultanas, half the almonds, the dill, chickpeas, and half the cauliflower. Cover the tin with a double layer of foil, sealing well, then bake for 30 mins until the rice is tender and stock is absorbed.

- STEP 5

Fluff up the rice with a fork, then fold in the remaining cauliflower (this creates a contrast of cauli textures). Scatter over the extra dill, the remaining almonds, the pomegranate seeds, if using, the pickled red onions and remaining lemon wedges to squeeze over.

Quinoa, pea & avocado salad

Ingredients

- 100g frozen peas

- juice 1 lemon

- 2 tbsp olive oil

- ½ small pack mint, leaves only, chopped

- ½ small pack chives, snipped

- 250g pack ready-to-eat red & white quinoa mix (we used Merchant Gourmet)

- 1 avocado, stoned, peeled and chopped into chunks

- 75g bag pea shoots

Directions

- STEP 1

Put the peas in a large heatproof bowl, pour over just-boiled water, then set aside.

- STEP 2

Pour the lemon juice into a small bowl and whisk in some seasoning. Keep whisking as you slowly add the olive oil, followed by the mint and chives.

- STEP 3

Drain the peas and tip into a large serving dish. Stir in the quinoa, breaking up any clumps. Pour over the dressing, then fold in the avocado and pea shoots. Serve immediately.

Spicy salmon tabbouleh

Ingredients

- 400g bulgur wheat

- 500g salmon fillet, pin-boned

- 3 tbsp sunflower oil

- 2 onions, finely chopped

- 5cm piece ginger, peeled and finely chopped

- 2 tbsp curry paste (we used korma)

- 300g Greek yogurt

- juice 1 lemon, plus 2 cut into wedges, to serve

- 300g smoked salmon

- handful coriander or parsley, roughly chopped

Directions

- STEP 1

Cook the bulgur wheat in plenty of salted water for 7 mins (or follow pack instructions). Drain, tip into a large bowl and leave to cool. Put the salmon fillet on a foil-lined grill, brush lightly with oil and season. Grill for 7-10 mins, turning halfway, until the fish flakes easily. Cool.

- STEP 2

Heat the remaining oil, add the onions and ginger, and fry for about 5 mins until softened and lightly coloured. Stir in the curry paste and cook for 1 min, stirring. Remove from the heat and stir in the yogurt, lemon juice and some seasoning. Leave to cool.

- STEP 3

Skin and flake the salmon fillet. Cut the smoked salmon into strips. Add the fresh salmon and half the smoked salmon to the bulgur wheat with the dressing and half the coriander. Stir everything together lightly, so as not to break up the salmon flakes too much. Tip onto a serving platter and scatter over the remaining smoked salmon strips and coriander. Add the lemon wedges and serve.

Warm mackerel & beetroot salad

Ingredients

- 450g new potato, cut into bite-size pieces

- 3 smoked mackerel fillets, skinned

- 250g pack cooked beetroot

- 100g bag mixed salad leaves

- 2 celery sticks, finely sliced

- 50g walnut pieces

For the dressing

- 6 tbsp good-quality salad dressing

- 2 tsp creamed horseradish sauce

Directions

- STEP 1

Boil the potatoes for 12-15 mins until just tender. Meanwhile, flake the mackerel fillets into large pieces and cut the beetroot into bite-size chunks.

- STEP 2

Drain the potatoes and cool slightly. Mix the salad dressing and horseradish sauce together in a salad bowl and season. Tip in the potatoes – they should still be warm.

- STEP 3

Add the salad leaves, mackerel, beetroot, celery and walnuts, and toss gently. Serve with crusty bread.

Courgettes with mint & ricotta

Ingredients

- 2 tbsp olive oil

- 2 tsp unsalted butter

- 4 large courgettes (we used a mixture of green and yellow), sliced

- zest and juice 1 lemon

- pinch of chilli flakes

- 70g ricotta

- extra virgin olive oil, for drizzling

- handful mint leaves, picked and roughly chopped

Directions

- STEP 1

Heat a large, heavy non-stick frying pan or cast-iron skillet over a medium heat. Heat 1 tbsp of the oil and 1 tsp butter together and add half the courgettes in one layer. Cook for 2 mins, then turn the heat down to medium-low and cook for 5 more mins untouched, until the underside has a nice colour. Flip the courgettes, then grate over some lemon zest, pour over half the lemon juice and season with salt, pepper and chilli flakes. Cook for a further 5 mins or until very tender. Repeat the process with the remaining slices of courgette.

- STEP 2

Transfer to a platter and top with spoonfuls of ricotta. Drizzle over some extra virgin olive oil and scatter over the mint to serve.

Stir-fried greens with fish sauce

Ingredients

- ½ head Savoy cabbage

- 125g purple sprouting or Tenderstem broccoli

- 2 tbsp groundnut oil

- 4-6 garlic cloves, finely sliced

- 75g baby spinach

- 2 tbsp fish sauce, plus extra for seasoning

- 1 tsp caster sugar

Directions

- STEP 1

Remove any discoloured or coarse leaves from the cabbage, then halve it. Remove the hard central ribs and discard them, then shred the leaves. If using purple sprouting broccoli, halve any thicker stems lengthways.

• STEP 2

Heat the oil in a wok. Stir-fry the broccoli for 1 min, then add the garlic and cabbage and cook until the garlic is a pale gold colour. Quickly add the spinach and fish sauce and turn the veg over – the moisture should come out of the spinach and boil off quickly. Add the sugar and toss the vegetables again, then add a little more fish sauce, if you like.

Fish o'leekie

Ingredients

- 1 leek, finely sliced

- 500ml vegetable stock

- 300g basmati rice

- 500g cod or haddock fillet, skinned and cut into large chunks

- handful parsley, roughly chopped

- finely grated zest and juice 1 lemon

Directions

- STEP 1

Put the leek in a large microwave dish with 4 tbsp of the stock. Cover the dish with cling film, pierce the film with a knife, then microwave on High for 5 mins.

- STEP 2

Uncover the dish, then stir the rice and remaining stock into the leek. Re-cover with cling film, pierce and microwave on High for another 10 mins, stirring halfway through until the rice is very nearly cooked.

- STEP 3

Gently stir in the fish chunks, cover the dish with cling film again, then pierce and cook for a further 5 mins until the fish flakes easily and the rice is tender. Stir in the parsley, lemon zest and juice. Leave to stand for 2 mins before serving.

Chapter 5: Lifestyle Strategies and Beyond For Managing SLE

Coping and support

If you have lupus, you're likely to have a range of painful feelings about your condition, from fear to extreme frustration. The challenges of living with lupus increase your risk of depression and related mental health problems, such as anxiety, stress and low self-esteem. To help you cope, try to:

Learn all you can about lupus. Write down any questions you have about lupus as they occur to you so that you can ask them at your next appointment. Ask your doctor or nurse for reputable sources of further information. The more you know about lupus, the more confident you'll feel in your treatment choices.

Gather support among your friends and family. Talk about lupus with your friends and family and explain ways they can help out when you're having flares. Lupus can be frustrating for your loved ones because they usually can't see it, and you may not appear sick.

Family and friends can't tell if you're having a good day or a bad day unless you tell them. Be open about what you're feeling so that your loved ones know what to expect.

Take time for yourself. Cope with stress in your life by taking time for yourself. Use that time to read, meditate, listen to music or write in a journal. Find activities that calm and renew you.

Connect with others who have lupus. Talk to other people who have lupus. You can connect through support groups in your community or through online message boards. Other people with lupus can offer unique support because they're facing many of the same obstacles and frustrations that you're facing.

Exercise and physical activity recommendations

If pain or fatigue—or both—have you struggling just to get through the day, working out is likely the last thing on your mind. But exercise, especially gentle strength training, can improve some lupus symptoms.

Strengthening your muscles helps prevent joint weakening and damage. It also helps counter fatigue and lupus-induced lack of energy.

Benefits of low-impact exercise for lupus

You can build a stronger body and have more energy—no gear required! Low-impact exercises are effective and are less stressful on the body.

This type of exercise has a low injury risk, making it safe for people who have balance problems and numbness of the hands or feet. Once you get the green light from your doctor, try the routine below, designed by Kim Truman, a National Academy of Sports Medicine–certified trainer in Dallas who has trained people with lupus.

The exercises are designed to boost both lower and upper body strength. This workout will also improve mobility and lessen joint pain. If any exercise is too challenging, simply follow the "take it easy" variation.

Fit in five

Twice a week, do 8 to 12 repetitions (reps) of each exercise in order. Then repeat the entire series once or twice more. It's OK to rest for a few minutes between each set of reps.

1. Squats

Stand with feet hip-width apart and arms extended at shoulder height in front of you. Bend knees as you sit back. Rise up to the starting position and repeat.

TAKE IT EASY: Start the move standing in front of a chair; sit down instead of squatting.

2. Alternating lunge

Stand with feet together and hands on hips. Take a big step forward with the right foot and bend your knees. Rise up as you step back to the starting position. Repeat, stepping forward with the left foot, then return to the starting position. That's 1 rep.

TAKE IT EASY: Grasp a table or the top of a chair for support.

3. Incline pushup

Take a big step back from a countertop and grasp the edges with hands shoulder-width apart. Bend elbows, bringing chest toward the counter. Push up, extending arms to the starting position, and repeat.

TAKE IT EASY: Do the move with your hands pressed against a wall.

4. Reverse crunch

Lie on your back on the floor or a yoga mat. Bend knees and place feet on the floor; extend arms straight down on the floor beside you. Slowly bring knees toward your chest, lifting hips slightly, then lower legs to the starting position and repeat.

TAKE IT EASY: Raise one knee at a time, alternating legs.

5. Bridge

Lie on your back on the floor or a yoga mat. Bend knees and place feet on the floor; extend arms straight down on the floor beside you. Lift hips until your body forms a line from knees to chest; hold hips up for 5 seconds, then lower to the starting position and repeat.

TAKE IT EASY: Don't lift your hips as high and eliminate the hold.

Alternative therapies and their role in managing SLE

Sometimes people with lupus seek alternative or complementary medicine. There aren't any alternative therapies that have been shown to alter the course of lupus, although some may help ease symptoms of the disease.

Discuss these treatments with your doctor before initiating them on your own. He or she can help you weigh the benefits and risks and tell you if the treatments will interfere adversely with your current lupus medications.

Complementary and alternative treatments for lupus include:

Dehydroepiandrosterone (DHEA). Taking supplements containing this hormone along with conventional treatment may help reduce lupus flares. dehydroepiandrosterone (DHEA) may lead to acne in women.

Fish oil. Fish oil supplements contain omega-3 fatty acids that may be beneficial for people with lupus. Preliminary studies have found some promise, though more study is needed. Side effects of fish oil supplements can include nausea, belching and a fishy taste in the mouth.

Acupuncture. This therapy uses tiny needles inserted just under the skin. It may help ease the muscle pain associated with lupus.

www.ingramcontent.com/pod-product-compliance
Lightning Source LLC
Chambersburg PA
CBHW071827210526
45479CB00001B/23